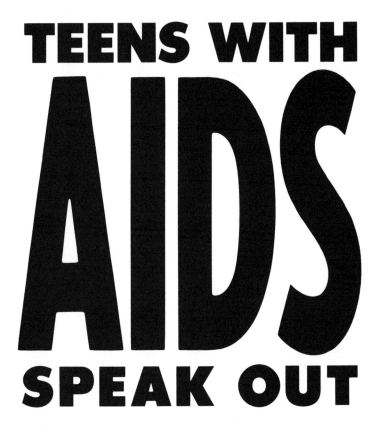

TEENS WITH AIDS SPEAK OUT

TEENS WITH AIDS SPEAK OUT

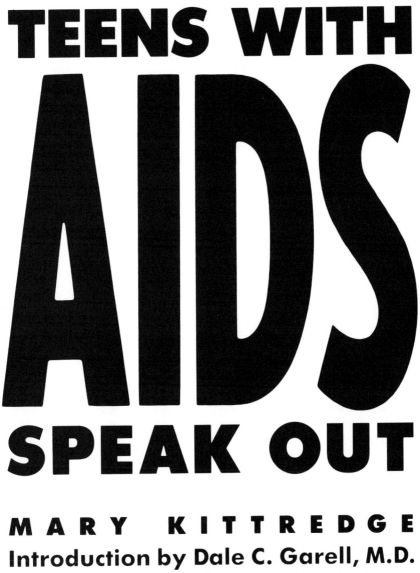

MARY KITTREDGE

Introduction by Dale C. Garell, M.D.

Co-Chairman, 5th National Pediatric AIDS Conference

JULIAN Ⓜ MESSNER

Julian Messner

JULIAN MESSNER and colophon are trademarks of Simon & Schuster,
Inc.
Design by Michael J. Freeland.

    10 9 8 7 6 5 4 3 2 1   lib ed.
    10 9 8 7 6 5 4 3 2 1   paperback

Library of Congress Cataloging-in-Publication Data
Kittredge, Mary.
    Teens with AIDS speak out / Mary Kittredge ; introduction by Dale
C. Garell.
      p.   cm.
    Includes bibliographical references and index.
    1. AIDS (Disease) in adolescence.   I. Title.
RJ387.A25K58 1991
362.1′9697′9200835—dc20   91-26562
    ISBN 0-671-74542-5 LSB   ISBN 0-671-74543-3 (pbk.)   CIP

*To the young adults who so generously shared
their time and experiences with me,
this book is dedicated with hope and affection.*

CONTENTS

INTRODUCTION

Dale C. Garell, M.D.
Co-chair, Fifth National Pediatric AIDS Conference

By now, you have probably learned a lot about the AIDS epidemic—from school, from reading about it in the newspaper, from TV programs and movies about people with AIDS. You probably know that it is caused by the HIV virus, transmitted through exposure to blood and blood products as well as by sexual contact with an infected individual. You probably also know that there is no known cure, but that many promising treatments can help reduce complications and prolong life. And you might know that adolescents are increasingly at risk to acquire AIDS because many young people are being exposed to the virus.

A few of you may even have known somebody with AIDS and have had the experience of living with the illness. If so, you understand the realities of caring for these people, who have one of the most medically complex and socially devastating illnesses in this or any century.

But for most of you who read this book, AIDS is mostly about abstract facts and very little about people with AIDS. And, because young people are now only beginning to tell their own AIDS stories, there is very little understanding about how AIDS affects teenagers.

This book is about real stories of real kids who have been experiencing this epidemic firsthand. Some of the stories are likely to move you deeply. Others will make what has been until now an academic experience a very real opportunity to learn about how AIDS affects teenagers.

The book is not written to scare you or to raise a series of "shoulds" or "should nots" that adults frequently preach to young people ... this approach has never worked well anyway. Rather, this book is about you—your choices and your lifestyle—and some very real issues for you to consider about your own behavior and about you as a caring, concerned individual who may one day have to deal with AIDS in your own circle of friends or family.

For sure, the AIDS epidemic is not going away. And researchers talk about teenagers being the next major group at risk of contracting AIDS. So a book like this is increasingly likely to be important to you as you experience young adulthood.

Now, what do we know about influencing behavior? Actually a lot about what works, but not very much about what might work for *you*. We know that it doesn't help to moralize or try to force a change in anyone's behavior. We know that knowledge alone isn't enough. We also know that the more real we can be without scaring you, the more likely you will be to consider what the message is: that you have some clear choices about your own behavior, that your sexuality and sexual experiences are individual decisions, not something imposed on you by the people around you, and that being responsible for your own actions is what life at its fullest is all about.

So it is my hope that you will read this book—to learn a little more about AIDS and HIV infection in teenagers, to examine the very real questions it raises about how you live your life, and most important, to help you make some decisions about yourself. Only you can prevent the spread of AIDS. So take a few moments to rid yourself of any previous biases and beliefs about AIDS, have an open mind and heart, and take care.

PREFACE

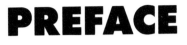

"Those who cannot remember the past are condemned to repeat it," wrote the great philosopher George Santayana. He meant that if we look back at our errors, and at the misfortunes they have caused us, we may be able to prevent those things from happening to us all over again; but that if we ignore our mistakes, the very same disasters will continue to afflict us. For example:

In May 1982 there were only about 700 people with AIDS in the United States, most of them homosexual men.

Health officials were very concerned, but to the average person AIDS meant little. Not much news about it was in the papers or on TV. Among the millions of people in the United States, after all, 700 did not seem like many. And besides, AIDS was happening only to "other people"—mostly to homosexuals. AIDS was too bad for the unlucky ones who got it, most people believed, but it really wasn't a big problem.

That way of thinking, of course, was an error. And because people didn't think *they* could get AIDS, many didn't protect themselves by avoiding behaviors that spread it. The result:

Just nine years later, by May 1991, the disease that was not supposed to be a big problem had killed more than 110,000 Americans. An estimated 1 million more were infected. The toll in human suffering was ghastly, both for people with AIDS and for their loved ones. The financial costs rose into the tens of billions of dollars. AIDS was, by all accounts, a disaster.

Also in May 1991, about 700 American teenagers had AIDS. Health officials were very concerned, but to the average person the information meant little. Not much news about it was in the papers or on TV. After all, 700 teenagers didn't really seem like very many. Besides, most people thought, AIDS happened only to "other kids"—teens who were drug addicts, or had sex with strangers, or in some other way had "brought it on themselves." AIDS was too bad for the unlucky teens who got it, most people believed, but it really wasn't a very big problem.

Sound familiar? It does to the young adults who shared their stories for this book, because for them the deadly history of AIDS has already begun to repeat itself. Like most young adults, Christina, Jim, Mike, Dawn, Krista, Peter, and David didn't think they could get AIDS—but they did. In *Teens with AIDS Speak Out* they tell how they became infected and what it's like to live with the disease. They comment on their hopes for the future; the difficulties of being a person with AIDS at home, work, and school; the medical treatments they undergo in order to stay alive; the pain and sorrow the disease has caused them; and the way they face the real probability of their own early deaths, because AIDS is virtually universally fatal. They also talk about how other teens can avoid going through what they are going through.

Why do they speak out? Because, more than anything, teens with AIDS want two things: they all want a cure, so that they can go on living. And they all want what's happened to them *not* to happen to *you*.

The young adults who appear in this book are real: none of them are "made up" characters. They are living proof that AIDS can happen to anyone—to me or to you, right now— the way it did to them. We can not yet cure AIDS, but we can grant the other wish of the young adults who speak out in this book: we can listen to them, learn from their experience, and by doing so, avoid repeating history.

Thanks to all who assisted me in writing this book: Karen Hein, M.D.; Larry DeAngelo, M.D.; Wally Brewer, Regina Robinson, Scott Walker, Jean Genasci, Terry Taylor, and the staff and volunteers of the clinics, outreach groups, support centers, and health organizations who gave information, referrals, and much encouragement. Everything that is correct in this volume is due to their excellent help; if errors remain, they are my own.

ONE

A
HISTORY
OF
HEARTBREAK

"**W**hen my baby got sick," says Dawn Marcal of those first terrible days of her three-month-old daughter's illness, "the doctors asked me if I used IV drugs. And I knew what they meant. I said 'Oh, my God, you don't think she has *that,* do you?' I was still calling it *that* at the time. I didn't even want to say the word. Later, of course, we started calling it AIDS."

Dawn knows she became infected with the virus that causes AIDS when she was about seventeen. She wants her real name used in this book because she works to educate young adults about AIDS, and she feels that being open about herself helps people to understand better—about AIDS, about people who have it, and about how to avoid getting it.

"I had used a variety of drugs as a teenager," Dawn recalls. "I had tried a lot of different things, crazy things. I had sex with guys, too."

Dawn didn't know it when she was seventeen, but at that time sexual contact and sharing needles used to inject IV drugs were two of the main ways a terrible new disease was being spread. It had first been noted early in 1981, when otherwise healthy young men in New York and California began dying from a strange illness doctors had never seen before.

People who became ill with the new disease had fevers and swollen glands, lost weight, and suffered from infections; they had skin cancers called Kaposi's sarcoma, a condition so rare that many doctors couldn't identify it at first. The cancers spread fast, and the young men became seriously ill with a kind of pneumonia called *Pneumocystis carinii,* which healthy people weren't supposed to be able to get.

Overall, it seemed that the victims' immune systems— the system in the body that fights illness and infection— were breaking down. No one knew where the problem came from, or what caused it. No one knew if it was contagious (if people could spread it to one another) or was the result of some toxic substance in the environment; all doctors and scientists really knew was that a lot of young men were dying of it.

Dawn's own story began at about the time the illness was

first being recognized, in May 1981, when she was fifteen. A disease, however, was the last thing on her mind. "All I really wanted to do was find a wonderful guy, fall madly in love, and have a wonderful, romantic relationship. The big mistake that I made was when guys said to me, 'Hey, Dawn, if we have sex it will make our relationship stronger,' and I believed them. So I would have sex with them. But instead of bringing us closer it created a whole new set of problems, and I would end up getting hurt. It took me a while to figure out that ninety-nine percent of the time that was what would end up happening, so I kept on getting emotionally hurt."

Meanwhile, doctors at the federal Centers for Disease Control in Atlanta, Georgia, had become interested in the new illness. As more cases appeared, they realized that most people getting sick were homosexual men. The doctors began to wonder if something about some homosexuals' living habits made a person likely to get the new disease: perhaps some homosexuals used some new toxic, illegal drug doctors didn't know about, or something about the sexual practices of this group was causing the illness.

Dawn and her friends, however, did not know about the new illness at all; few people did. Not even doctors knew for sure whether it could be spread from person to person, or if so, how it might spread. Teens like Dawn certainly had no way of knowing that they might be vulnerable to it. Besides, Dawn had other problems on her mind.

"I decided that to avoid getting hurt I was going to build a big wall around my feelings," she says. "No one was going to know how much I was hurting inside, and I pretended I didn't know either. And while I was in that stage I tried all kinds of drugs and alcohol. When I was seventeen, I tried IV drugs [the kind people inject into their veins], and to do that I used shared needles."

While Dawn was trying to bury her unhappiness in experiments with drinking and drugs, two scientific developments sped medical investigation into the new illness. First, a few scientists, including Dr. Luc Montagnier of the Pasteur Institute in Paris, had already been studying a special kind of virus called a retrovirus.

(A virus is a tiny organism that does not do anything but invade cells of other organisms. Inside an invaded cell the virus takes over the machinery the cell uses to reproduce; now, instead of making more cells like itself, the invaded cell makes millions of new virus particles. The new viruses burst out of the cell, killing it, and then go on to invade yet more cells where the process is repeated. Some common virus-caused diseases are chicken pox, the common cold, and herpes simplex, which causes cold sores.

A retrovirus is a special kind of virus that contains a chemical called reverse transcriptase. Reverse transcriptase enables the virus to imitate the cell's instructions for reproducing itself so that the virus can become part of the cell. This changes the cell permanently. Later the virus uses the changed instructions to make more viruses.)

Because retroviruses can infect the immune system cells of people, some doctors thought such viruses might be causing the new disease. But if that was so, the ailment could be contagious—a frightening idea. In 1919 another contagious viral illness, a particularly bad form of influenza (the "flu"), killed millions. Just as worrisome was the fact that virus-caused diseases cannot be cured with drugs such as antibiotics; this is why there is, for instance, no cure for the common cold. Scientists began to worry that a new virus-caused illness was killing people, and that it might be spreading fast.

The other scientific advance that occurred in the early 1980s was the invention of a device called the Fluorescent Activated Cell Sorter. Only since 1980 had the National Cancer Institute had the new machine, which cost $500,000. With it, immune-system cells in a person's blood (called T-cells) could be counted swiftly and automatically; before this, such cells were counted slowly by a trained technician peering at them through a microscope.

Doctors already knew that in people sick with the new disease, T-cell counts were out of whack; their blood contained fewer of the cells that fight disease, called T-4 cells, and more of the ones that tell the body to stop fighting disease, called T-8 cells. In 1981 Dr. Jim Goedert at the National Cancer Institute used the cell-counter to do T-cell counts on fifteen apparently healthy homosexual men. Half the men had very abnormal T-cell counts. This discovery showed that the new disease was already more widespread than anyone thought, and it made finding the cause—and a cure—even more urgent than before.

Dawn's own life, though, remained unaffected by any of these developments—or so she thought. In fact, as time passed life seemed to improve a lot for her. "Because," says Dawn, "a funny thing happened: I grew up. I quit doing drugs. I finished high school, and went to college for a while. I got a wonderful job. And I met a really great guy."

For Dawn, it seemed the "bad old days" were all behind her. What she had dreamed of—but thought she couldn't have—was happening. "I was ecstatically happy," she recalls.

Doctors and scientists, however, grew more unhappy—and more worried—as the picture of the new disease grew more complex: Starting in 1982, a few people from Haiti had begun getting sick, along with a few people who had used illegal IV drugs. A few women also became ill. Doctors wondered what in the world homosexual men, IV drug abusers, women, and people from Haiti could possibly have in common to make them all susceptible to a single ailment. What was going on? And more worrisome—how bad would the situation get?

By 1984, just as Dawn's future seemed to be brightening, more facts had appeared: Many of the homosexual men who got the new disease had more sexual contacts with more different people than did homosexual men who had not gotten ill. The men who got sick also told doctors that, during sexual contact with other men, they were the receptive partner (the one whose body was entered by the other's penis) more often than men who did not get ill. Doctors found that having sex with a lot of different people and being the receptive partner in sexual contacts tended to make a homosexual man more likely to get the disease. But that did not explain how IV drug users, women, and Haitians were getting it.

Meanwhile, at age nineteen Dawn had become concerned about the events of her earlier teen years, but not because of AIDS. "I guess I was a little defensive about my so-called sordid teenaged past," she says, as she recalls how worried she was that her new love would reject her if he found out about the things she had tried. "So I sat this guy down and said, 'Hey, look, I've done all these different drugs, and I've had sex with this number of guys,' and I went through all the things I'd done in the past. 'And if you can't deal with any of this,' I told him, 'then you'd better just get the hell away from me.'

"And he just laughed. He said, 'Dawn, don't be so defensive. You were a teenager. You did crazy things. All teenagers do crazy things. So did I.' I was very relieved. Soon after that, we got married."

What Dawn did not know was that scientists had now found the ways the new disease was spreading. By the time Dawn got married, it was known that the illness was contagious, caused by a virus, and was being spread by two main fluids of the normal human body, fluids commonly transferred from one person to another either during sex or when needles were shared by drug users.

The first fluid was semen: the fluid the male's penis releases during sexual climax (when a person "comes"). This was the way the illness was spreading among homosexuals and to some women with the ailment so far: via sexual contact. They had been the receptive partners during sex with someone who was already (and probably unknowingly) infected with the ailment; semen entering their bodies was carrying the disease.

The second human substance that could spread the illness was blood. With this knowledge, the whole picture of the disease began to make a lot more sense. When an infected person's semen entered another person's body during sex, the virus causing the illness was getting into the uninfected person's bloodstream: by tiny tears in the skin inside the rectum or vagina, or sometimes through sores or other breaks in the skin of a man's penis or a person's mouth.

When a person who used illegal IV drugs injected the drugs, he or she might not use a clean needle; if the needle had been used by someone with the ailment, a small amount of the infected person's blood got into the bloodstream of a person who, until then, had been uninfected. Again, the culprit was the direct contact between the infecting virus and the person's bloodstream.

These facts meant that, because of her sexual activities and IV drug use in the past, Dawn was at serious risk of having the virus that causes AIDS. They also meant she could pass it to her husband or to any children she might have. Unaware of the danger, however, and already taking care of her husband's three-year-old son, Christopher, Dawn wanted a baby of her own. Six months after she got married, one of her fondest dreams came true: she became pregnant, and was even happier than before.

In the scientific community, more about the illness called AIDS was becoming known. In 1984 Dr. Montagnier and Dr. Robert Gallo of the National Cancer Institute had each identified the specific infecting virus (then called HTLV-III virus or Human T-Cell Leukemia Virus, now called HIV, or Human Immunodeficiency Virus) that brought on the illness. Yet the ailment, although a matter of urgency to doctors and scientists who realized how terrible the disease already had become, was not of much interest to "ordinary" people even by 1985. As far as most of the general public knew or understood, only homosexual men and IV drug users were getting the new disease. This caused many people to dismiss the idea that they might get it themselves. And because many people disapproved of homosexual men and of drug abusers, they didn't care very much about the people who *were* getting it.

Dawn didn't suspect it could have anything to do with her, and she certainly didn't think it could affect her baby, whose birth she and her husband awaited with growing excitement. "I thought being pregnant was just the most wonderful thing in the world," she remembers now. "Every time I felt the baby move I got so excited. It seemed to me like just the most amazing thing. I never got tired of it."

Among some people, however, awareness of AIDS *was* growing. Among homosexual men, the death toll from it was rising fast, and they knew the illness was being spread by certain kinds of sex acts, especially by rectal intercourse (in which one person's penis is inserted into the other's rectum). They realized that using a condom (a thin flexible sheath over the penis) during sexual intercourse helped protect people from exposure to the virus. And they knew that oral sex (in which one partner's mouth comes in contact with the other's penis or rectum) could also transmit the virus via even very tiny breaks in the skin, nicks or scratches too small to see or feel.

Thus homosexual men began to practice "safer sex": more and more men wore condoms, and many of them avoided sex acts such as unprotected oral sex that could put one person's blood or semen in contact with another's vulnerable skin. As a result the rate of new infections began dropping in this group. But among heterosexuals the story was different. Believing that "only homosexuals got it" or "only drug addicts got it," people who did not belong to one of those groups did not feel the need to practice "safer sex." The fact was that sex between men and women could transmit the virus; more easily from men to women because the man deposits potentially virus-bearing semen into the female's vagina during sexual intercourse, but also from women to men, since secretions in the vagina may also carry the virus into broken skin on the man's penis. Oral sex between men and women or between women and women might transmit the virus also, if either partner had any broken skin or open sores in the mouth or on the genitals.

For people who were not drug addicts, but who "experimented" with drugs only once in a while, the situation was similar. Even sharing a needle just once with a person carrying the virus could infect a person. But these facts were not widely understood, and many people also thought they could tell who might have the virus just by looking at them, and avoid having unsafe sex or sharing a needle with infected people. On top of that, the idea that "my friends couldn't have the virus—only those *other* people could have it" remained widespread.

As a result, when Dawn's baby was born, no one thought the new baby's health problems could have anything to do with AIDS. "When Lindsey was being born she swallowed some fluid that got into her lungs," Dawn says. "Then she developed pneumonia and had to be in the hospital for a week. At last, though, she got better and went home, and everything seemed fine.

"We had about three months of normal babyhood," Dawn goes one. "Every time she did something new I just got so excited. If she blew a spit bubble, I was delighted. I loved being a mom, I just adored it all. But I noticed that if she would cry hard, she got a little blue around the mouth. The doctors said there was nothing wrong at first, but after they saw it happen, too, they put her in the hospital. They thought it meant she didn't have enough oxygen in her blood and they wanted to find out why."

The doctors at the hospital said Lindsey had pneumonia again but they didn't know what was causing it. That was when they asked Dawn and her husband if they used drugs. If so, Dawn might have gotten the virus that causes AIDS via IV drug use, passing it to her baby before birth. That could explain the pneumonia.

"Of course I automatically said no about drug use, because we didn't use any drugs," Dawn remembers. "And then we kind of forgot about it for a while—only, not for long. Lindsey got somewhat better, but she didn't really thrive or gain weight. And she never *really* recovered completely from the pneumonia."

At that point, Dawn started thinking hard about the doctors' questions concerning drug use. She realized that even though she didn't do those things now, in the past she'd had experiences that could have exposed her to the AIDS virus: unsafe sex and IV drug use with shared needles.

"I thought I couldn't possibly have the disease. I'm strong and healthy, I never get sick, I have no symptoms—that's what I thought. But on the off chance that I did have it, I needed to know for the baby's sake," Dawn says. "So I figured I'd better go for the AIDS blood test."

By 1985, a test to detect AIDS antibodies (particles that show a person's body has been exposed to the HIV virus and has tried—unsuccessfully—to fight it off) had been developed by scientists. Dawn says having the test was simple: a small amount of blood was drawn from her, to be tested. But waiting the two weeks for the results was emotionally very difficult.

"Two really terrible weeks," she recalls. "And I prayed so

hard during that time. But my result came back positive."
Even though she had no symptoms, her blood carried antibodies to the virus that causes AIDS, which meant she had
the virus. Lindsey's blood also tested positive; before the
baby was born the virus had passed from Dawn's bloodstream to that of her child. Dawn's husband was also tested,
but he turned out not to be infected.

"In that way," said Dawn, "we were lucky. It's like playing
Russian roulette: you can have sex with a person who has the
virus a lot of times and not catch it, or you can have sex with
an infected person just once—and catch it. Fortunately, my
husband hadn't caught it." Still, that was practically the only
fortunate thing about the whole situation.

Dawn's parents knew she had been tested and that her
test had come back positive. "My parents and I are very
close, and from the first they've been completely supportive.
When we found out the test results, though, I said to them,
'Don't tell anyone else. I don't want anyone pulling back
from the baby or treating her badly because of this.' But my
mom said 'No, Dawn. We're going to tell *everyone*. And if
people can't handle it, they can just stay away from us.' I said
okay, and from that point on we told all our families and all
our friends."

Other family members' reaction to the news was varied.
"My dad told his parents," she says, explaining that he left it
up to his parents whether or not to inform the rest of that
side of the family. "But they decided they didn't want to tell
their other relatives, and we didn't push it. And then last year
there was a big article on us in the paper with pictures of us
and everything. So my dad called his parents and said, you'd
better tell the family because this article is going to be on the

front page, and they might see it. They said okay, that they would tell them. But they didn't tell them, and after the article came out I had aunts and uncles calling up, and calling my dad, of course wanting to know what the hell was going on. That was pretty bad. My dad's parents got some pretty heavy flack from their other kids for not telling them sooner. They wanted to know; they wanted to be able to offer their help and support."

Dawn goes on: "And then I got some weird reactions, too. One relative sent me a birthday card, which he'd never, ever done before. Another one brought me a present, and I hadn't seen the girl in five or six years. Sometimes it's like, 'Oh, now *I* know somebody with AIDS. Somebody in my *family* has AIDS, and they're gonna *die*.' And they feel like they want to get close to you before that happens."

She hasn't faced any outright hostility toward herself or her family on account of having the virus. And even if she did, says Dawn, "Hey, the worst thing that could possibly happen to me has already happened. What do I care if people don't like me?"

By "the worst thing," Dawn means her infant daughter's illness. For the next year and three months after they found out the baby had AIDS, Dawn and her husband did everything they could to save Lindsey and to make her life as happy and comfortable as possible. They gave her the anti-AIDS drug AZT, which was then used in children only experimentally. It still is the only drug known to slow the progress of the disease. They gave her vitamins and took her to a variety of specialists. They battled desperately in every way they knew against the disease that threatened Lindsey's life.

By that time, a lot of other people were battling it, too.

The Centers for Disease Control in Atlanta say that by the end of 1987 more than 67,000 cases of AIDS had been diagnosed in the United States alone. More than 38,000 had already died. Scientists were working desperately to develop a vaccine to prevent more people from getting the virus, while they continued to test one new drug after another in the hope that something more effective than AZT could be found.

Attempts to learn the origins of the virus were made as well, in case that knowledge might lead to progress in the fight against the ailment. Several questions needed to be answered: Was AIDS a virus that had always existed, but had mutated (changed) and suddenly become deadly? Was AIDS a disease that had spread from animals to people? This theory was based on the fact that there is a similar disease, called Simian AIDS, that afflicts some monkeys. Or was the virus an entirely new germ?

The answer to these questions remains unknown, although the virus has been found in frozen blood samples from as early as 1963. So doctors know the virus was already beginning to infect people nearly thirty years ago. Scientists think the disease may first have appeared in Africa, where it is a severe health problem—in some parts of Africa one in three people is sick or is carrying the disease—but again they are not sure.

Meanwhile, efforts were made to educate people about AIDS in the hope they would avoid the risky behaviors that could spread the ailment. In some parts of the country, these efforts were opposed on moral grounds: talking frankly to young adults about sex and drugs might encourage them to try these activities, some people worried. Likewise, when some health workers began giving clean needles to drug addicts so that the addicts would not become infected through shared dirty needles, some people said this encouraged drug abuse. Nevertheless, although "safe sex" education and "no dirty needle" programs were slow in gaining acceptance, they continued in many parts of the nation and have almost certainly saved lives.

But none of that was enough to save Dawn's baby girl. In 1989, when Lindsey was only eighteen months old, she died of the illness Dawn had gotten unknowingly as a teenager, and passed just as unknowingly to her child. "Yesterday was the anniversary of my daughter's death," Dawn says softly. "She was my whole life, everything I lived for. I loved her so much. And yesterday, I went to the cemetery and put flowers on her grave."

In 1983, when Dawn herself became infected, just under 4,400 people were known to have AIDS in the whole country. By early 1991, more than 3,000 new cases were being diagnosed in the United States each *month*. The CDC estimates that more than a million Americans may carry the virus; like Dawn, who has already had one bout of AIDS-related pneumonia, most will become ill and many—perhaps most—will die. CDC experts say that, like Dawn, many were probably infected as teenagers. A CDC estimate says that thousands of teens may be infected—carrying the virus without knowing it or having symptoms—in addition to the nearly 700 cases diagnosed among teens by early 1991.

The 700 diagnosed cases may not sound like many, although for each of those young adults and his or her friends and family the diagnosis is a tragedy. But these young adults know they have the ailment, and knowing they carry the virus keeps most of them from pursuing risky behaviors such as unsafe sex and sharing needles to inject drugs by which they could infect other people.

The thousands of silently infected young adults do not know, and neither do their friends. They look fine and feel healthy; it is absolutely impossible to distinguish them from anyone else. In fact, they are just like everyone else except for two things.

First, their lives are in serious danger from the disease, and second, they can give the virus to anyone with whom they have unsafe sex, or with whom they share a needle to inject drugs. A person with the AIDS virus can be the quarterback of the football team, captain of the debating squad, class clown, the prettiest girl in the school. He or she can be fat or thin, black or white or Spanish or Asian, rich or poor, popular or unpopular, nasty or nice, very religious or not religious at all. He or she can be homosexual or not, a drug user or not, a straight-A student or not. The virus doesn't care about any of those things. AIDS is an equal-opportunity disease. All it needs to infect a person is one shared needle or one act of unsafe sex.

"So," says Dawn, "what I tell people now is that whether it's unsafe sex or IV drugs, the few minutes of pleasure you can get from those things are not worth the years of pain that you can also get from those things. Also, when I was trying IV drugs and having unsafe sex with people, it was at a time when I didn't think I was tall enough, or smart enough, or pretty enough, or whatever it was that made me feel bad about myself. That didn't mean I had to go and do things that would harm me, or let other people lead me into those things, but I did. My point, when I talk to other people about it, is that they don't have to repeat my mistakes. They don't have to have something from their past come along and kick them in the butt, just when they've finally found happiness, the way it did to me."

Today, Dawn takes the anti-AIDS drug AZT regularly, although she cannot take it all the time because the drug's strong side effects have damaged her liver. She's careful about what she eats and visits her doctor at least once a month for tests and checkups. It's vitally important for her to try to avoid catching the "everyday" illnesses most of us could fight off without trouble; for Dawn, because the AIDS virus has damaged her disease-fighting immune system, such illnesses could be fatal. And she knows that there is still no cure for AIDS, so like many other young adults with the disease Dawn faces a future clouded with uncertainty.

TWO

WHAT
IS
AIDS,
ANYWAY?

"**I** got AIDS by having unsafe sex with a friend when I was fifteen years old," Jim S. says. "See, sex is something that, when you're young, you do partly to help establish your identity, your individuality as a person. And at one time I thought, 'Why not?' People should be free to have all the sex they want."

AIDS stands for *Acquired Immune Deficiency Syndrome*. It is a disease that is *acquired:* something a person gets, rather than something he or she is born with. It affects the *immune system.* When the immune system cannot defend the body, we say it has a *deficiency:* it does not work as well as it normally should. And AIDS causes a *syndrome:* a group of symptoms or harmful conditions that are often fatal and are recognized as going along with AIDS.

Jim looks up earnestly. He's a handsome, red-haired young man of twenty-three with a quick intelligence and a ready grin, a "boy-next-door" type dressed casually in a sweater and slacks. He speaks easily and laughs often, sometimes tipping his head to think a moment before making a comment or answering a question.

"But I don't feel the same way about it anymore," he goes on, "because there's a very serious sexually transmitted disease going around now, and it can kill you. It's not just some story to control teenagers and scare them away from having sex. It's a life-or-death thing and it's real. People need to know that. And they need to know that if they're going to have sex, then they must protect themselves against this disease."

On the floor nearby, Jim's black cat Max is playing while Jim speaks into a tape recorder for this interview. Jim jokes that the cat should write its own book entitled, "My Owner Has AIDS." It's funny—when Jim makes a joke it's hard not to laugh, because he's naturally witty and fun to be with—but it's sad, too. It's hard to think about a person as delightful as Jim—or any young person—having AIDS.

"I grew up in a strongly religious family, in a small town," Jim says. "I attended church every Sunday, I was an altar boy, and I went to a Catholic high school." Jim did not think that a teenager from an ordinary community, someone with a good family, strong values, and a religious upbringing, could possibly get the virus that causes AIDS. He especially did not think he could get it from another teenager like himself. But he could, and he did, because the virus that causes AIDS can infect absolutely anybody.

Jim's real name is not being used here because some of his family and friends do not know he has the ailment. "I want to decide for myself whom I will tell, and I want to tell them myself, not have them learn it from a book," he says.

Some members of his family also do not know that Jim is homosexual, living in a long-term relationship with another young man, Art, whom he loves. Jim has known he has AIDS only for a short while; of course, it came as a terrible shock to him and to Art, who does not have the virus. Jim and Art are in many ways still struggling with the knowledge of how the virus has changed their lives, and that it could end Jim's life.

"I basically just kind of crashed into this," he says of the disease and the sudden way it struck him. "I had this cough, and I thought I had bronchitis. I went to see the doctor, who said that I had pneumonia and should have the HIV test (the test for antibodies to the AIDS virus). The test came back positive on a Thursday; on Monday I went into the hospital because my pneumonia had gotten so much worse. So it all really happened so fast: one week I felt perfectly fine, and the next I was extremely sick."

Health professionals are very concerned that AIDS can spread easily among teens—that they can become infected while still in high school, as Jim did—because this is a time of life when people struggle to establish their independence, their selfhood, and their sexual identity. It is a time when people want to be accepted in their own group—to be "in," not "out"—and to love and be loved. And it is a time of pressure: from parents, teachers, friends, and even one's own feelings.

A girl may decide to have sex with her boyfriend because she feels she loves him, or because she fears she will lose him if she says no. A boy may decide to have sex because he knows sex feels good or in order to prove that he is mature. Either one may feel too embarrassed to suggest using a condom when they have sex. And either may decide to try drugs because friends will call them "chicken" if they don't, or in order to defy parents who want to "tell them what to do all the time," or because being "high" may seem to help ease painful feelings of unsolved problems in their own lives.

Experimenting with sex or drugs has never been a very wise thing to do, but until recently these activities have been among the risks many young adults commonly took. The results could be very painful and damaging: an unwanted pregnancy, a drug arrest, a sexually transmitted disease. In the worst case, a girl might die while having an illegal abortion. A young adult might also die of a drug overdose or in an alcohol-caused accident. Still, these instances were relatively rare; most young adults might be "wild" for a while, but the vast majority of them survived their risky experiments and grew up to lead long, happy, and productive lives.

But about ten years ago the virus that causes AIDS began causing the disease in larger and larger numbers of people, and all that changed. Today, a young person who has unsafe sex just once or tries IV drugs just once, can get the incurable disease called AIDS and wind up facing death at an early age. The risky act doesn't have to be with a stranger or a "bad kid" or an older person. AIDS can be carried by a person's best friend. It's terrible, and it's not fair, but it's true, as Jim discovered when he became ill.

"I was in the hospital for eight days," he says. "And when I first went I was in a bad way: I was shaking, had a temperature of a hundred and six, coughing, and I couldn't breathe. But the hospital was completely full so I had to wait in the emergency room until there was a bed and a room for me. That was one of the few times I broke down and cried: first when my doctor told me my test was positive, that I had the AIDS virus. And then when I went to the hospital and waited for two and a half hours there, with a temperature of a hundred and six, having a lot of trouble breathing. I was very sick, and I was frightened."

Today, four months after he learned of his illness, Jim has recovered from pneumonia and returned to college part-time. He wants to earn a degree in social work; he also works part-time at a family planning clinic. But he hasn't forgotten how seriously ill he was, or how hard the experience was on him and Art.

"I told myself that I was really sick, and this was just something I needed to do to get better," Jim remembers, "but that attitude is hard to keep up when you're just *so* sick. It worked for about an hour and a half, and it was even harder on Art, who was waiting there in the emergency room with me, the poor guy, but then I started to lose it, kind of falling apart emotionally as well as physically, and poor Art, he was just climbing the walls, seeing me feeling so awful, wanting to take care of me but not being able to do anything. At one point he said to me, 'I just want to take you home.' "

Jim knows it is not the virus itself that makes AIDS dangerous, but rather the other diseases that can overwhelm his body now that AIDS has damaged his immune system. Right now, for example, Jim has a painful cold sore on his lip. It is caused by a virus called herpes simplex. A person without AIDS would find it at worst an inconvenience, but Jim's cold sore isn't going away by itself. It hurts, and he is using an expensive anti-viral cream called Zovirax in the hope that it will go away eventually. If it doesn't, it could spread to his throat or other parts of his body. For Jim, a little thing like a cold sore could turn into a serious problem, because Jim's immune system is running at less than one-third its normal power.

Jim frowns briefly, remembering the pneumonia again. "Once I got admitted to the hospital, things got a little better," he continues, "and everyone in the hospital was very helpful. But I did have to have some painful tests. One was an arterial blood gas test, which is to find out how much oxygen is in your blood. It really hurts, and I had to have that a couple of times. I had to wear an oxygen mask. I had three IVs (tubes that deliver medicine through a needle directly into the bloodstream). And for the first four days I couldn't even walk, I was so sick."

The immune system consists of a wide range of organs, tissues, cells, and chemical substances that work together to defend the body against illness and infection. Its key ability is *recognition:* it can tell the difference between material that belongs to the body and material that does not.

A second immune-system ability is *specificity:* it can tell the difference between two similar materials, and decide that it should fight off one but not the other.

The system's third main ability is *memory:* once it has

recognized and fought off a certain kind of foreign organism or substance once, the immune system will recognize and fight that foreign material even faster the next time. The medicines Jim received against his pneumonia fought off the illness, but they did not fix his damaged immune-system abilities.

"After a while I improved," Jim says. "But the thing was, improvement did not mean I was cured. This pneumonia meant I didn't just have the virus. It meant I had full-blown AIDS, in which you can get lots of different diseases. My immune system was not going to get better. And when you're a young guy like me, never even been in the hospital before and learning you have a potentially fatal condition—well, it's very hard."

In Jim's case the virus had silently been present in his body for eight years before it became active. For him, pneumonia was the first sign of the virus's effects and its threat to his whole future.

"I have a lot I want to do in my life, and now I know that I might not get to," Jim says quietly. "And when you're young and something like this happens, you haven't yet had a lot of life's good experiences, life's high points, to balance it off."

This is one aspect of AIDS that is particularly cruel: that a person can become infected without even knowing it—by doing something that might be unwise but that a person shouldn't have to die for—while still in high school and not even find out he or she is infected with the virus until a couple of years later, when it has already done severe damage to his body. But it happens. It happened to Jim, and it is the way AIDS happens to many of the teenagers who get it.

"My doctor doesn't even do a T-four cell count on me

when I go for my checkups anymore," Jim says (T-4 cells are cells that turn the body's anti-infection defenses "on"). "Because by the time I got pneumonia, my count was already under two hundred. Normal is from about six to twelve hundred. My immune system is pretty wiped. And they're not going to come back all the way, my T-4 cells, not with any of the treatments available now. I take the anti-viral drug AZT and that slows the virus down, but it doesn't stop it, and it doesn't get rid of it. There isn't any drug that can do that."

Scientists don't know for sure what triggers the virus that causes AIDS to "wake up" in a person's immune system and begin doing harm, but once it does, a person's T-4 cells can be nearly destroyed very quickly. Now Jim gets out his bottle of green-and-white AZT capsules. This drug, the only one approved to slow the progress of AIDS, is extremely expensive: a bottle of one hundred capsules currently costs $144, and Jim uses up a bottle every three weeks. In the spring of 1991 the Food and Drug Administration was trying to lower the cost of AZT. Because a government scientist originally developed the chemical zidovudine that is AZT's active ingredient, the FDA says that other companies—not just its current manufacturer, Burroughs Welcome—should be allowed to sell it. Such competition would drive down the drug's price. At current prices, however, Jim's AZT alone will cost more than $2,000 per year.

In addition Jim must have regular checkups, X-rays, blood tests, and other drugs, including one called pentamadine, which is a mist he inhales into his lungs to keep his pneumonia from coming back. The pentamadine costs nearly $200 each time he takes it. If he gets any other infections or complications from AIDS, those will have to get costly treatment as well. In short, staying alive with AIDS costs money: a lot of money.

"I have a good health insurance policy as one of my benefits at the clinic where I work," he says, "so insurance has covered all my medical costs so far: it has paid my hospital bills, for example. But it does have limits; it pays for only two thousand dollars worth of prescriptions per year and of course my medicines will cost more than that. So whatever the extra is, I'll have to pay for. And as a student with a part-time job, I don't make much money."

Not all young adults or their families have insurance, and a person with AIDS can need tens of thousands of dollars' worth of medical treatment every year. These people may use up savings, lose their homes, and have to go on welfare. A person with AIDS who becomes too sick to work may lose not only his or her job, but the insurance benefits that go along with it. As a result, about 40 percent of people with AIDS, including young adults with the disease, now depend on government-financed programs such as Medicaid to pay their medical bills. The cost of the programs has risen from about $10 million in 1983 to nearly $700 million in 1991, in part because of the cost of AIDS.

But to qualify for Medicaid, a person must be very poor *and* be over sixty-five, or a member of a family with children, or completely unable to work. This means that if a person with AIDS has no health insurance, or loses the insurance because he or she has become too ill to work, then he or she might not be able to get any medical care at all until it is nearly too late for treatment to do any good. If Jim S. gets too sick to work at the clinic, he could become one of these people. He probably won't, because his friends and family who do know of his condition love him and can and will help him. But not all young adults with AIDS have such support from family or friends.

Congress is considering laws that would provide health care to such people before they become desperately sick. But as of early 1991, such laws had not yet been passed, and the $600 to $700 million they would provide is not enough to care for all who need it now, much less the thousands of new cases of the disease that doctors are expecting to see in the United States by the year 2000. Money for doctors, nurses, medicines, treatments, even the light, heat, and phone bills of hospitals that will care for all these newly sick people has to come from somewhere, and so far our nation has not yet figured out where.

In addition to medicines and treatments, young adults who have the AIDS virus need a lot of encouragement and help to deal with the disease. "It's unbelievably time-and-energy-consuming just staying on top of all the things you need to do: get your medicines, take your medicines, cope with the side effects of the treatments, have your checkups, figure out your insurance forms, pay your medical bills—it goes on and on. And it's not as if you're spending all this energy on something good. You're doing it on account of something rotten," Jim says, "and that makes you feel even worse about it all."

He feels fortunate to get as much help as he does. "Besides friends and my family I also get a lot of support from the people in my church," he reports. "I don't know what I would do without them. When I was in the hospital they called and visited me all the time. When I got home they called and brought food. I knew they prayed for me, too, and it was all just so helpful."

Deciding whom to tell that he has AIDS has been a complex issue for Jim. "Of course I told Art," he says. "And I told one good friend of Art's," he goes on, explaining that this was so Art would have someone he could talk to about it besides Jim. "But then I got so sick so fast that I just had those two people tell my other friends, who also go to my church. I knew I needed big-time support; no way I was going to get through this alone."

Informing his parents of his situation was particularly hard for Jim. He faced this task while he was in the hospital. "I really did not know what to do about that. I was critically ill, and it looked like I would be in the hospital a long time. So I called my father and asked to speak to my mother, but she wasn't there. So I said, 'I really don't know how to tell you this but just to tell you.'" Then Jim told his father that he had tested positive for the virus that causes AIDS and was now seriously ill with an AIDS-related pneumonia.

Jim's father told his mother about the situation, and both of them called Jim back. "That was a rough conversation," says Jim. "One of the hardest parts was talking about telling my brother. I'm pretty close to him, and I was going to call him. But my father said, 'Don't call him. This is a really hard thing to learn about on the phone.' And then he kind of choked up and just couldn't go on. It was a very tearful phone call."

Jim eventually did tell his brother about his illness. But there are still people whom he has not told, whom he would like to tell. "It's hard for me, because when I tell it, it's as if I have to live it all over again." He understands that people have to go through their own sorrow for him, but he is trying to go forward with his life and doesn't want to be dragged back into an earlier stage of dealing with having AIDS.

"For example, when I got home from the hospital people would call me, and be crying and crying on the phone. And I don't want to go through that too much with people. There are only a few people whose reaction I'd actually be worried about though [in the sense that they might be afraid they could contract the virus by casual contact with him]. One person that I work with, I'm concerned that she might feel weird about things like sharing food. Maybe I'm not giving her enough credit, but that's my gut feeling so I'm going to go with it."

One thing that's happened since he learned he had AIDS really makes Jim's face light up. "I made a new friend, my first new friend since I found out I had the virus. And that's really super. I started talking to this guy standing in a line with me at school registration. He showed me around the campus, we had lunch together the next week. Meanwhile here I am, my life has just been completely changed, and I'm wondering how can I get to know someone new. How can I make a new friend and not tell him about what's happened to me, about something so important in my life? But it's much harder telling someone new than someone you already know."

In discussing their classes, Jim found a way to tell his new friend that he had AIDS. "We were talking about some classes we were in, and I said to him that I'd started taking some of them before, but I'd had to drop out of school for a while because I'd been sick, and I'd been in the hospital. And he said, do you mind if I ask why? So I told him I'd had pneumonia, and there was this little silence. And I went on to say that one of the results of my being sick is that I take these—and I took out my bottle of AZT. He recognized them, and he knew that meant AIDS, and his reaction was to say that he had a lot of friends who take AZT. I said it was kind of hard for me to talk about, because it had all just happened recently. And he put his arm on my shoulder and said he was really glad that I'd told him. And I thought, Wow! A post-diagnosis friend. It was a big step for me," Jim finishes, clearly pleased that he has not only kept his old friends, but has retained the ability to make new ones.

Still, he says as we near the end of our conversation, there is one thing about being a *young* person with AIDS that makes some kinds of support more difficult to get: most other young people with the virus don't yet know they have it—and unless they get tested, might not know for years—so Jim has no one else his own age who also has AIDS with whom to share his feelings and experiences.

"It's hard," he says. "I'm tired of being the baby with it, always the youngest one. I went to one meeting for people with the virus, where everyone was older than me. And not only was nobody else my age, but no one was even talking about having the virus. I wanted to say 'Look, let's talk about this. What's going on with your lives; how are you dealing with this?' But I didn't want to be the one to start. So it was a little weird. I felt a little lonely, uncharacteristically shy. I'm going to go back to that group, I think. But I'd just like to talk this all over with someone who's young like me and who also has it, you know?"

THREE

IT
HAPPENED
TO
ME

"I didn't think I could get AIDS," says fifteen-year-old Mike W., who became infected with the virus when he was thirteen. "Sure, I'd heard of it, but that was about all. It seemed so distant. Even after my doctor sent me to get tested, I didn't really worry because I was so sure I didn't have it. At age thirteen I thought I knew a lot. But then the test results came back positive, and it all just kind of blew up in my face."

Mike is a tall, blond teenager who lives with his father

33

and brother in a small town in a southern state. His father and mother are divorced. He's a sophomore in high school, a near straight-A student who enjoys snow skiing and volleyball, and also likes to go to the beach. He wants to go to college, and after that he's interested in becoming an underwater archaeologist, to explore sunken ships and find their treasure.

"There aren't a lot of jobs in that field," he jokes. "I'm thinking of maybe becoming an underwater repair specialist first; they do welding and that kind of thing. And with some experience I could go on to the more exciting stuff. Meanwhile, I'm pretty much the same as any other teenager. I go out with my friends, I do my share of experimenting in life, but I don't take it to the lengths some people do, like experiments with sex or IV drugs."

One of the ways Mike resembles most other teens is that his thoughts and feelings about sex are not completely settled. In his case this includes the fact that on some days he feels more attracted to males, and on others he's more attracted to females.

Scientific surveys of young adults say that as many as 37 percent of young men in the United States may have sexual contact with another male at least once during their teen years. "But it's hard, having these feelings," Mike says. "First, for me, there's the confusion that one day I'll feel one way— I see a neat guy and feel like I'll want to be with him—and then the next day there's a girl who's really nice, and I feel like in my life I want the wife, the kids, and the dog and the white picket fence, you know."

On top of his own feelings, Mike doesn't want to disappoint his dad. "Of course, my dad wants me to like girls. I know he feels that way. He'll say, 'Hey, look at her, isn't she cute?' So I feel like . . . well, I know that's what he'd like. And then I have to deal with the kids in my school."

Mike pauses, sorting out his thoughts. "In school, if you are a guy and you act the slightest bit homosexual—if you talk a certain way, or you walk a certain way—the other kids call you a fag. You get teased, you get beat on. So I am learning to act really straight. A girl walks by, I'll say, 'Hey, she's hot,' just like the other guys do. And there's a guy in class, he does act homosexual, and I tease him just like the others do. I feel like I have to do it. It keeps the teasing away from me."

Mike doesn't like hiding part of his real personality from his friends, but he feels he must. "I do enjoy going with my father on some trips outside our small town," he says. "Then, where no one is looking at me, I can act more like myself. But in school and with my friends, all I can say is that it's hard."

Mike has also had an experience that complicates the whole issue of sex for him. When he was thirteen, he became involved in a sexual relationship with a man twenty years older than himself. Mike's feelings about this relationship led him to tell his father about it. But Mike did not want to reveal the man's name, because he knew if he did, the man would be prosecuted for having sex with a minor (a person under the age of eighteen).

For an adult to touch a person Mike's age in any sexual way is a very serious crime; what Mike had been thinking of as a relationship was really, in the eyes of the law, a case of child molestation. It was also a very serious risk to Mike's health, although Mike didn't realize that at the time.

"I had asked him if he had any diseases I could catch,"

Mike recalls, "and he told me no, he didn't. He did say his former partner had AIDS but that he didn't have it himself. He said he had leukemia but that I couldn't catch it. When I think of it now, well, that did seem a little weird, but I believed him." Unfortunately, the man did have the AIDS virus and he transmitted it to Mike via sexual contact.

Still, Mike didn't get the virus *because* he had sexual contact with another guy, or *because* the person he had sex with was older. The fact that Mike is a good guy himself did not protect him from the virus, either. Mike got the virus that causes AIDS because the person he had sex with happened to have it and didn't wear a condom while he was having sex with Mike. Having unsafe sex with *anyone* who is infected is one main way of getting the virus, as Mike discovered later.

The first hint that something might be wrong arrived a few months after the relationship with the man had ended: Mike came down with a flu-like illness that his doctor couldn't identify. "My doctor thought it might be chicken pox or mononucleosis," Mike remembers, "but they tested me for those, and I didn't have them. And then whatever it was just kind of got better by itself."

Hearing that Mike had had unsafe sex, however, the doctor then advised Mike to have the AIDS antibody test. Mike didn't take it very seriously, and his first test was negative, but his doctor was still very concerned about him. The reason: sometimes a person can have the virus for a while—doctors are not sure how long this "latent period" is, but in most people it is probably a matter of weeks or months—before the test can show it.

About one in twenty AIDS-infected people do not make antibodies against the disease at all, even though they have the virus; these people can have the infection without ever getting a positive reaction on all but the most advanced AIDS tests. They can also pass it to others. Some who get infected have illnesses that resemble "flu" or other ailments, as Mike did, shortly after they get the virus; the majority, however, never have any sign of becoming infected. These people, too, can spread the ailment to others. None of them "look sick." Only people in the last stages of the disease show any outward, ongoing signs of illness.

"A few months after my first AIDS test," Mike says, "I had a physical exam required for sports at school. The doctor had me tested for AIDS again and this one came back positive." That is, the repeat test showed there was a strong chance he had the virus. His father had been asking him to tell the name of the person with whom he'd had unsafe sex, but Mike had refused; he was worried that the man—who had been living in the same house as his aunt when Mike visited her—would get in trouble.

"And then I started thinking," Mike says. "Here I was with the virus, and I knew this guy had given it to me. I'm not sure if he lied to me about having it or maybe he was trying to deny in his own mind that he had it. Maybe he said he had leukemia so that if he ever had to go to the doctor he could say his symptoms were from leukemia and not AIDS. But whatever his reason was for telling me he didn't have it, the truth was that he did. I knew he was still out there, probably having unsafe sex again like he did with me, probably giving the virus to other people. So then I did tell his name. The police arrested him; he admitted what had happened; and now he is in jail."

Mike pauses. It was difficult for him to give the name of a

person he once considered a good friend. It's hard for him to think that someone he thought really cared for him might in fact have been lying to him, possibly taking advantage of him. And it is hard, no matter what the reason, to think of someone he once considered a friend being in jail now. The whole experience has brought Mike a lot of pain and sorrow, a lot of mixed feelings even aside from his concern for his health, and it's not easy for him to talk about it. Still, he shares what's happened, hoping someone else might read about it and get some benefit from it, so that what has happened to him will not happen to others.

"If I had to give advice to other people my age," he says quietly, "I'd have to say stay away from sex until you're older if you possibly can. Whoever it might be with, even someone in your own school, wait until you are old enough to handle all the stuff that goes with it, really. Because what goes with it is a lot more than you think. But if you do have sex, then it's got to be safer sex, and don't let anybody tell you different because I know what I'm talking about. You can't expect the other person to protect you. You've got to protect yourself."

Mike pauses a moment, then goes on in a brighter tone: "What I'm really glad about, though, is that my doctor was smart enough to put it together and have me tested. I mean, this is a small town and AIDS is not something you necessarily think about. But he realized it wasn't just something that happens in cities, or to drug addicts or older people. He knew it could happen to me. And if he hadn't been thinking that way we might have forgotten about it. Then I would not have gotten treatment right away. I could have gone on for six or eight years, or until I got really sick. It's better for my health that I found out early. They know now that taking the drug AZT can postpone symptoms in some people with the virus, so I take AZT."

Mike also thinks about the possibility that, if he hadn't found out he had the virus, he could have given it to others. "I wouldn't have known I had it. Who knows how many people I could have given it to? I could have just gone on spreading it without ever knowing it."

Mike is absolutely right on both counts: if he hadn't gotten that strange illness, or if his doctor hadn't been so alert, he would not have been tested. That could have been a disaster for Mike. When he got the results of his positive AIDS test, his T-4 cell count had already decreased to just over 200 (normal is about 1,000) due to the effect of the virus.

But today, after months of taking the anti-viral drug AZT, Mike's T-4 cell count has risen; he feels fine and has had none of the infections that tend to strike people whose immune systems are crippled by the virus. And he has not passed the virus to anyone, as he might have had he not learned he had it himself.

Still, he knows his life remains at risk from the disease. Today he feels fine; tomorrow he might not. There is no way of getting rid of the virus once it is in a person's body.

"See, that's why everyone has to be so careful," Mike says. "One thing I've already decided about anyone I might ever get involved with in the future is that before we get to the point of possibly having sex, I'm going to tell the person I have the AIDS virus. Even though of course it would be safer sex [sex with a condom does not *guarantee* protection against the virus that causes AIDS, but it lowers one's chances of getting the virus], I believe the other person deserves to know. But listen: not everyone is always going to be that honest. And not everyone is even going to know *they* have it. If I hadn't been tested, I wouldn't have known. That's why everyone has to use condoms, every time."

Having the test itself, Mike says, was a simple thing. "You go to the place where they're doing the tests anonymously," he says. "That means you don't have to tell your name. Instead, they assign you a number. They take a little blood, and that's no big deal, either. Then a few days to two weeks later, you go back and tell them your number, and they tell you your result. That's it. You never have to tell your name. Even if the test is positive—well, if that happens you get counseling, right away you can get help, but your name still doesn't come up."

After a person has had blood drawn for an AIDS test, it is sent to a special laboratory. There, technicians check it to see if it contains AIDS antibodies (a sign the person's immune system has tried—unsuccessfully—to fight off the AIDS virus). To do so they use a technique called an ELISA (Enzyme-Linked Immuno-Assay) test.

But the ELISA test is not perfect. Some people get a positive reaction, indicating that their blood carries the virus, when they really don't have the virus that causes AIDS. Instead the positive results are due to other factors in their blood. A positive test in a person who does not have the virus is called a *false positive*. People who test positive are given a more sensitive test called the Western Blot test, which can rule out other factors and reveal whether they really do have the virus.

Also, some people who do have the virus will receive a

negative result on the ELISA test. A negative result in a person who really has the virus is called a *false negative*. A false negative can occur because the immune system of the infected person cannot make antibodies against the virus. Or it may be that, as in Mike's case, the person's immune system simply hasn't had time to make antibodies against the virus. He or she will likely test positive for the virus later, as Mike did. A person who has symptoms of AIDS-related illnesses, but tests negative on the ELISA and Western Blot tests, can receive a third, even more sensitive test that will definitively identify the presence or absence of the virus in the blood.

"After I tested positive, I had several more tests to make sure I really did have the virus," Mike says. "Just to make sure the positive test was not a mistake, or just some weird reaction. But I found out it wasn't a mistake. I wish it had been, but it was real."

Mike goes on: "Anyone who's had unsafe sex or shared needles for IV drugs should go and get tested." He says this because a young adult with the virus needs treatments that can slow the onset of symptoms, while one who doesn't have it can (1) stop worrying, and (2) avoid getting it by steering clear of risky behaviors.

Mike also believes a young person who goes alone for the test should tell his or her parents right away if it comes back positive, even if that also means telling them other things they will not like, such as that one has had unsafe sex, experimented with IV drugs, or has homosexual feelings.

"I mean, my dad has been right there for me since he found out about all this," says Mike. "He does a lot of the work that has to be done on account of my having the virus, like finding out what I need, keeping up on new treatments, staying on top of things. I don't see how a person my age could do it all, alone."

But, he says, there are exceptions: if a young adult thinks his or her parents will react very badly to hearing that a person wants to be tested or has been tested, then he or she could seek counseling, and ask the counselor to be present when this news is given. A counselor can help everyone—the young adult and his or her parents—in this difficult but necessary conversation. A young adult whose parent has been violent in the past, or who thinks a parent might really kick the young adult out of the house, for example, should definitely consider seeking the help of a counselor. Then the counselor can help the young adult talk with the parent about AIDS testing.

Learning that a young adult has the virus is emotionally very difficult, both for the young person and for his or her family. So people who test positive receive ongoing counseling to help them understand and deal with this information. Mike W.'s father was with him when he received the positive results of his second test. The news was upsetting to both of them, although to Mike it didn't seem real at first.

"When my test came back positive my dad put his arms around me and cried," he says. "But at the time all I could think was, 'How gross, get away from me. Just get me out of here.' See, we'd never been all that close, and all of a sudden he puts his arms around me."

Immediately, Mike and his father began to receive counseling to help them deal with their feelings, as well as to cope with the practical problems they would now be facing. They were given information about the virus, referral to a doctor who specialized in treating it, and answers to their questions. Now, two years later, Mike has not felt any symptoms from the virus, so he does not worry too much about it. "I pretty much just take it a day at a time," he says.

For now, for Mike, that's enough. But even two years after he first learned he had the virus, he and his father still attend counseling together to help them handle their feelings. And Mike attends a support group made up of other people who have the virus. Like other young adults interviewed for this book, however, he reports that he is the only teenager in his support group, so sometimes the discussions there don't have a lot to do with his daily life. And like other teens with the virus, he wishes he had someone his own age to talk to about it: someone like himself, who is going through what he goes through.

"They mostly talk about work," Mike says of the group he now attends, "about how hard it is to keep having the virus a secret from people they work with, and things like that. I haven't told a lot of people I have the virus, but I've told a few. I haven't had any bad reactions."

Mike's father feels it's best not to tell very many people that Mike has the virus. Maybe some people would be accepting, he thinks, but others might not—and he doesn't want to risk getting a hostile or fearful reaction from people. Mike also feels that not telling people he has the virus allows him to "get away" from thinking about it; at school, for instance, he can forget about it and just feel like any other teenager.

"I'm not keeping it a strict secret the way some are in my support group, though. There's this one kid I told, and I still see him around school. Actually, the people who do know, maybe about seven people, have been really nice about it. So anyway I don't have some of the problems the older people in the support group have. Money and insurance—my father takes care of those things."

Yet Mike feels any support is better than none. "It still helps me," he says, "just being around other people who have the same thing I have. It makes me feel like I'm not the only one."

In fact, Mike is definitely "not the only one." If everyone in the United States were tested, 1 to 1.5 million would react to the Western blot test with a positive result, says the CDC. Of people in their early twenties who have actual symptoms of AIDS—there is no accurate count of people who are infected but have no symptoms—experts think most or even all became infected as teenagers. And experts on teenagers with AIDS agree that the problem of AIDS among young adults is growing fast.

One result is that, as time goes on, more young adults with the virus will be present in families, schools, and communities across the nation. And because fear of the disease is so common, many may face discrimination: in schools, work, housing, and other areas of daily life.

In the next chapters we will meet more young adults who have the virus that causes AIDS, examine the most common myths and fears about AIDS, describe how society has reacted toward people with the virus, and learn the specific scientific facts about how AIDS can spread and how it cannot, as well as how a person can avoid contracting the virus. In doing so, we will see that the virus that causes AIDS is indeed something to be feared, but that people who have it are just like ourselves and need not be feared at all.

FOUR

LIVING
WITH
AIDS

Not everybody with AIDS is dead, you know," says David Kamens, a twenty-year-old who became infected with the AIDS virus at age seventeen. "I'm living with this disease; there are a lot of people living with it; and because of misunderstandings and fears, many must live with it alone. There isn't enough support for people with AIDS, especially for young people, and because they're afraid of the reaction they may get, many have to keep that fact that they have the virus a secret." They are,

David feels, all alone when they need others most; it's something he's trying hard to change.

David is a slender, good-looking young man who grew up in a fairly well-to-do family in Connecticut. When he is not busy working to educate people about AIDS, he likes to paint, travel, ride his bicycle, and take his big, energetic dog out for walks. Always talented in the arts, by age fourteen David was a dancer in a near-professional-level ballet troupe. Even though serious dancing requires a lot of strength and skill, he was teased by some of his classmates for being more interested in dance and artistic pursuits than in "macho" activities such as competitive sports.

But in the performing arts, David found a group of friends who liked and accepted him. So although he was not accepted by some classmates, with the people he really cared about David was one of the "in" group. Looking back on it now, he feels it was partly to stay "in" with his friends that he began having sex in his early teens.

David was and is homosexual. This, however, is not the point: it wasn't having sex with other males that caused David to contract the virus that causes AIDS. Having any unsafe sex with anyone was what caused that. "I thought I had found role models," he says, "a peer group of people I could admire. But I really hadn't. I was putting myself in a lot of compromising situations. They weren't taking care of themselves. They weren't really being good to themselves. And I wasn't, either. I didn't realize then that I was important—that I was worth taking care of. And I didn't realize then that no one was going to take care of David except David. I was basically just going along with the crowd."

By 1986, when David was sixteen, he realized that having

unsafe sex had put him at risk for getting AIDS, so he had the antibody test. His result was negative: he didn't have the virus. After he learned this, however, he did not stop having unprotected sex. "I knew I wouldn't have AIDS; I knew my test would be negative. I felt like I *couldn't* get it, and in a way," he says, "finding out I really was negative felt almost like a license to go out and do even more unsafe things."

Doctors say this reaction is fairly common. Young adults who get a negative AIDS test may feel they must be "immune" to the disease—or that "good luck" and "thinking positive" can protect them. Or they may think that if they haven't got the virus yet then their friends must not be infected either; so it must be all right to go on participating in unsafe activities like unprotected sex with this "known" group.

Most of all, though, a negative AIDS test can encourage a person to go on believing a dangerous untruth: that AIDS can happen only to other people. A negative AIDS test can feel like "proof" that "it *can't* happen to me," when in fact it can happen to anyone. Someone who tested negative yesterday can do something unsafe today—and become infected while doing it.

That was what happened to David Kamens sometime between his first AIDS test, which was negative, and his eighteenth birthday. "A few months after my birthday I got really sick," he says. "I lost thirty pounds in three weeks and was in bed for two months with an infection called cytomegalovirus. It's an infection that is associated with having AIDS. A couple of months later I got the antibody test again."

That time, the test came back positive. "I kind of expected it would," he says, "because of that infection I'd had.

I pretty much knew the score by then. Still, I was only eighteen. Before I got sick I was thinking about taking the SATs, wondering which colleges to apply to, wondering where I'd be accepted—and then all of a sudden this happens."

As it turned out, David did not enter college that fall. He didn't go to college at all; instead, he began reading everything he could find on the ailment that had struck him. "I mean I read *everything*," he recalls, "about this thing I was living with." In the three years since, he has made it his mission to let other young adults know what he's learned: he travels to high schools and colleges to talk to students about the disease, and meets with lawmakers in Washington to work for more education to prevent AIDS and support for those who already have the virus. Meanwhile, David battles the ailment himself.

"I take eighty pills a day," he says. "Some are medicines that my doctor prescribes. Some are vitamins and nutrition supplement pills. Some are to prevent infections. I work hard on keeping my energies up. I'm careful about what I eat. I do everything I possibly can, and I try everything I think might work."

Still, it's an uphill fight: "I don't have very much of an immune system. My T-cell count is only about 30, so I get one infection after another. Right now I have thrush in my esophagus. [Thrush is a painful fungal infection of the tube that carries food to the stomach.] I see my doctor every couple of weeks. I've been in the hospital lots of times, for infections and for allergic reactions to medicines I have to take. It's not easy living with this thing."

David's experience also includes the fact that some people hate and fear AIDS so much that they hate and fear the people who have it, too—and he knows their hatred sometimes includes him. It is another reason why he works for a better understanding of the illness: because when people understand, they can protect themselves more effectively while reducing needless fear, hatred, and cruelty against people who have the virus.

"I've come out of a room where I've been giving a talk on AIDS," he reports, "and found the words "faggot, faggot," on the wall for me to read. It's because people still think AIDS is a disease only homosexual men get. When I've been in the hospital I've had my meals left out in the hall sometimes, because people wouldn't come into the room of a person with AIDS. I've had a doctor ask me rude questions about my sex life, questions that had nothing to do with my medical care. Those feelings, fear and anger, are because many people don't understand the disease."

David's experiences are not unusual. Many people with the virus, and some who are only suspected of having it, have had even worse things happen to them. In his book *AIDS in the Mind of America,* journalist Dennis Altman lists some of them: One man with the virus was rejected by his own family and not allowed to visit them anymore. Another told of a friend with AIDS: the friend's room in the hospital was left dirty, health care workers would not bathe him, the pilot of a plane taking him back to his home town to die did not want to transport him, and when he died the undertaker would not embalm his body; instead the workers at the funeral home poured the embalming fluid over him, wrapped him in a plastic bag, and sealed him hastily into his coffin that way.

Stories of needless cruelty and sorrow are seemingly endless: Altman tells of a divorced mother who refused to see or touch her children, who lived with their father who had AIDS. She was afraid she would get the virus from the children. In a park in San Francisco, twenty young adults attacked homosexual people with rocks and sticks, shouting, "Faggots got AIDS," and injuring several seriously.

In Florida in 1987, three young brothers who tested positive for the virus were rejected by their church, shunned by their whole town, and not allowed to attend school. But for the Ray brothers that was just the beginning.

These three brothers—Randy, Robert, and Ricky Ray—got the virus from blood products used to treat their hemophilia. In 1987, when they were ages eight, nine, and ten, word got around that they carried the virus. As a result, the barber wouldn't cut their hair. Their family got hate mail and threatening phone calls, and their school barred them from attending classes. After nearly a year of such treatment, a judge ordered the school to accept the boys—but when they went half the other children in their school didn't show up for classes. Those who did were briefly evacuated after a phoned-in bomb threat. But it was not until the family's house was burned down that the Rays gave up: they moved away.

"The children cried," said the boys' mother at the time, but they realized it was "for their safety." In their new school in another Florida town, the boys were accepted, and even received greeting cards of welcome from other students on their first day of classes. But their story is still one of lingering pain: as of early 1991 Ricky and Robert had both developed AIDS-related illnesses; only Randy is still healthy. And the Ray family does not have a "home town" any more.

Ryan White, a teenager who also acquired the virus

through treatments for hemophilia, was barred from his school in Kokomo, Indiana, in 1985 as a result of fear that he would spread the virus to other teens. Because of his hemophilia he couldn't play sports—even a small bump or bruise can be very dangerous to a person with hemophilia—so the isolation of being kept out of school was particularly hard for him. "I want to be with my friends like everybody else," his mother remembered him saying.

For all of 1985 his mother fought to give Ryan his wish, while some in the community tormented them both. Says writer Ann Marie Cunningham, coauthor with Ryan of his autobiography, in a 1990 *Ladies Home Journal* article, "The Whites were shunned, even in their Methodist church. The family got nasty anonymous letters, piles of garbage were left on their lawn, and someone even fired a bullet through their window."

In 1986 Ryan won one battle: under a court order, he returned to school. But the reception was not what he'd wished for. His classmates teased him unmercifully, made cruel jokes to his face, and wouldn't associate with him. Meanwhile he began having more serious AIDS-related illnesses. And he grew more afraid of dying—especially if he had to die in Kokomo, where people had treated him so badly. One day, out on a ride with his mother, he spotted a graveyard in the town of Cicero and said that when he died, he'd like to be buried there because it looked so peaceful.

In 1987, with Ryan's health failing, he and his mother moved to Cicero. He couldn't forget his illness and didn't really lose his fear of dying. Sometimes, his mother says, he couldn't sleep at night because he was thinking about it. But he had some fun, too—although he would have traded the fun if he could only have been just a normal, everyday teen-ager. "Like that," he once said, snapping his fingers. "I'd trade it just like that."

Instead, by 1988 Ryan White was perhaps the most fa-mous person with AIDS in the world, and numbered popular performers Michael Jackson and Elton John among his friends. He learned to drive the red Mustang Jackson gave him, had a part-time job, and attended the prom at his new school in Cicero. But as his AIDS progressed, he also got even sicker than before; by late 1989, his mother told Ann Marie Cunningham, "He had a hernia that made walking painful, but his [blood count] was so low the doctors couldn't operate. He got shingles [an infection of nerves and skin by the herpes virus] and sores on his legs that wouldn't heal. Often his throat was so sore he could barely whisper. Just taking a shower and getting dressed wore him out."

In March 1990, Ryan's condition began deteriorating fast, and after a week of lying unconscious and in critical condi-tion in an Indianapolis hospital, he died. Early in 1991 Ann Marie Cunningham published the book she and Ryan had written together: the story of a young man who wanted more than anything to be just an ordinary teenager, but who be-came instead a symbol of courage, hope, and love.

The struggles against ignorance and fear of AIDS that the Ray brothers and Ryan White faced have been repeated again and again across the country. Elisabeth Glaser, wife of the popular TV actor Paul Michael Glaser, contracted the virus through an infected blood transfusion in 1981. Even today with careful screening procedures for blood donors, there is still a small chance of getting AIDS from a blood transfusion. Organ transplants also carry a very small risk of transmitting the virus. But when Elisabeth Glaser received blood the chances of becoming infected from a blood transfusion were much higher. There was no test to detect the virus in donated blood as there is now. Elisabeth Glaser didn't even know she had the virus until after she had passed it to her two young children, Ariel and Jake. In 1988, while Jake remained symptom-free and Paul had tested negative, Ariel died of AIDS. But before that, the whole family went through seven years of hell.

"At first," she writes of the time when she was telling some of her friends she had the virus, "no one would allow their children to come and play at our house. Some friends refused to let my children come to their homes . . . some said their children could continue to play with mine, but only at the park. Some dropped out of our lives. The day after I told my yoga teacher about [our having the virus], she called to tell me she never wanted to see me again."

Rejection, pain, and heartbreak seemed to pile up impossibly high, and when her family needed an angel to help it get through, Glaser writes, "it seemed we had no angel watching over us."

After her daughter died, Elisabeth Glaser and two of her friends started the Pediatric AIDS Foundation to raise money for research against AIDS in children. So far, the foundation has raised more than $4 million, most of which goes directly into the study of pediatric AIDS. It also is working on a national emergency assistance plan for hospitals that treat children with AIDS, and conducts programs to help educate people about AIDS.

"Fifty percent of America is better educated [than when I learned my family was infected]," Glaser told an interviewer for *People* magazine in early 1991. "But if you're living next door to the other 50 percent it means nothing." She wants, she says, a kinder and gentler America not just for people who have power or money, but for all. Her book about her family's experience with AIDS is called *In the Absence of Angels*. In her work with the foundation, she is trying to supply the help of an angel her family did not have.

AIDS, very simply, is a hard thing for people to face and to think about—especially in connection with themselves. "There was a lot of alienation between me and my friends in high school when I first was diagnosed with the virus," David Kamens says, "because all of a sudden this disease was slapping them in the face, too. I haven't lost friends, but it's taken time [for them to get used to the idea]." Because David was very ill before he learned he had the virus, his mother and father knew he would be tested and knew the results were positive, so he never faced the task of telling them he had AIDS. "But my family didn't want to talk about it to other people for several months. And at the time I was angry about that: I wanted to tell people I had the virus, but they didn't."

But after a while, David's family felt more comfortable telling people about his condition. "My parents told people in their church. My brothers and sisters told friends. I realized people need time to come to their own understanding and have their own feelings, before they can talk about it. Now my family and I have gotten an incredible amount of acceptance and warmth. No one's thrown a rock through our window: just the opposite."

The negative reactions he's gotten—seeing hateful scrawls on walls, for example, at places where he has been speaking on AIDS, or being treated fearfully at times by hospital workers who do not understand the ailment—seem to have been more against the idea of AIDS than against David himself, and he doesn't take them personally. He feels self-esteem is a key to living with AIDS—as well as to avoiding becoming infected with the virus.

"I've worked hard to feel good about who I am today, so it just doesn't affect me too much," he says of the instances of negative reactions he's faced. "Before I got sick I was having unsafe sex, and I also drank and used drugs. I didn't have any understanding of the consequences. I didn't understand the value of life. Now, I really value myself and I value life. There's not much in life I take for granted. And if people react to me in a negative way, I know it's not because I deserve that kind of behavior. I know it's because of fear and misunderstanding about the disease."

When he first found out he had the virus, David went to a support group for others who had it. Like several others interviewed for this book, though, he found he was the only young adult in the group. Today, David gets his support from friends and family, and from his work helping other young adults learn more about AIDS. "It lifts me up," he says of educating teens about the reality of AIDS in their lives, and the dangers it poses to them.

"Two of my most important therapies are compassion and education," he goes on. "Education gives me hope that others will be able to avoid AIDS. And the compassion I get for my own situation from a lot of people I'm educating is something I can really draw on, myself. After I've come away from talking to young adults about AIDS, I really feel like I have some power. By supporting others in this way, I give myself support, too."

One of David's main messages to other young adults is that a person has the right to value his or her own life, and to decide to take care of it, no matter what the others are doing.

"No one ever said to me when I was fourteen, 'David, you are allowed to love yourself and to respect yourself, so you'll be able to live with choices that you make.' Now, I'm learning to live with the choices that I made, and with the consequences of those choices, but it's not easy. I hope others will get that message—that you're valuable, you have a right to take care of yourself, to not just go along with the crowd. You have a right to make healthy choices for yourself so you don't have to go through what I'm going through now."

David goes on: "We need more support for young people with AIDS in this country, and we need much, much more education about the disease, for everyone." Education will help keep more people from getting the disease, he feels, by making them aware of their own value and that they have a perfect right to avoid unsafe sex and other risky behavior, and it will help stop discrimination against people who have the virus, too.

Unsafe sex and blood-to-blood contact are the only ways a person can get AIDS. If you don't have sex at all, and you never share any hypodermic or other needles with anyone for any reason, and you don't have a blood transfusion or use other blood products, or get the blood of another person into contact with your blood in any other way, then your chances of getting AIDS are essentially zero.

If you only have safer sex (you use a condom *every single time*) and you *never* share hypodermic needles or have blood-to-blood contact, your chances of getting AIDS are also very low. The problem is that condoms can leak or break; if they do so during sex with an infected person, the virus can pass from one partner to another in the semen or vaginal fluids of the infected partner.

If you ever have unsafe sex, share a hypodermic needle with anyone, or have other blood-to-blood contact with anyone, no matter how healthy they look or how well you know them, you can get AIDS. The only exception is sex between two people who have both just tested negative for the virus and haven't engaged in *any* risky behaviors since being tested, who never share needles with anyone, who don't get blood transfusions or other blood products, and who *only have sex with one another—never with anyone else.*

You can *spread* the disease, without knowing you have it, by the kinds of sexual contact mentioned above or by letting someone else use a hypodermic needle you have already used. You can pass it to your unborn child, if you are a woman, without knowing you have it. You may be able to pass it to your newborn infant via your breast milk. If you are infected, you can *give* the disease to others by donating blood (but *you cannot get AIDS by donating blood*).

Those are the facts about how a person can get AIDS, or give it to someone else. But what about how you *can't* get the virus?

Luis Q., a sixteen-year-old who lives with his mother and sister in Massachusetts, doesn't have the virus himself, but his mother does.

"I have eaten from her plate," he says. "I have drunk from her glass. I hug her. I live right in the same house with her, and if you could get AIDS from things like that, then I would for sure have gotten it by now. But I haven't, because you can't get it that way. You get it from unsafe sex or blood contact, and that's it."

Luis is absolutely right. AIDS spreads in blood and via unsafe sex, and those are the only ways it spreads. That means you can't get it by sitting next to someone who has it. You can't get it if the person sneezes or coughs in your face. You can't get it from sharing toilet facilities with an infected person. You can't get it by hugging that person. You can't get it by babysitting for his or her children. You can't get it from that person's comb or brush, or even by using his or her toothbrush. You can't get it by living in the same house, apartment building, or even the same room with that person.

To get AIDS, you've got to have unsafe sex with that person, or share a hypodermic needle with that person, or have other blood-to-blood contact with that person, because AIDS spreads in blood and semen and that's *all* it spreads in.

Some people say that despite these facts, they would rather be "safe than sorry"—and avoid *all* contact with anyone who has the virus that causes AIDS. They want people with the virus to be kept out of schools, work, and anywhere they might have casual contact with uninfected people. Some even suggest people with the virus should have identifying tattoos, or that they be sent to an isolated place and made to stay there. Why is their over-cautious attitude not the proper course to take?

"I'll tell you why," says Luis. "Because it's wrong. First it's wrong on the facts: AIDS doesn't spread by casual contact. But also it's unjust. People with the virus need hugs and love as much as you do, you know. Maybe even more. My mom sure does. And another thing you should remember: you never know when you might need *them*.

"It's wrong to push a person away because they have the virus. To treat people with the virus with love and respect, the same as you would want for yourself—it's just the right thing to do, it's the way the world *should* be, that's all," Luis says.

But if the facts about AIDS are so plain, and the disease only spreads by blood or semen, why *are* some people so hysterical about the disease? Why do they burn down people's houses, scrawl hateful messages on walls, try to keep them out of schools and other public places, and do other terrible things to people who have the virus?

Of course, one of the reasons AIDS makes people so afraid is that it is often fatal. A deadly disease naturally causes fear; no one wants to get it. But along with the kinds of worries that people would normally have about a disease that can cause death, AIDS is also seen by many as being shameful—a "dirty" disease. The reasons are complex and have to do with what many people feel about sex, about morality, and about death.

Linking a disease to these feelings and then reacting in a "knee-jerk" way instead of thinking clearly and acting reasonably results in a stigma, a mark of shame associated with the disease and with the people who have it. Once a person has any sort of stigma, even though it is not deserved, he or she tends to be treated badly, with "automatic" fear, hatred, and discrimination, by the rest of society.

There are five main reasons why AIDS causes a stigma for those who have the virus. First, AIDS is a serious disease, and any serious disease tends to make people anxious by reminding them of serious diseases in general. Next, AIDS is often fatal, and the idea of death frightens people. Third, it is spread by sexual contact and in blood. Many people feel so uncomfortable about blood that they faint or become nauseated at the sight of it. Sex is also a topic that provokes a lot of very intense feelings in many. So a disease that is spread by these routes is bound to provoke strong feelings, too. Fourth, when AIDS first appeared in the early 1980s, homosexual men and drug addicts were identified as the "ones who are getting it." These two groups were already disliked by many people; the feelings of "they are bad" that people had about drug addicts and homosexuals "rubbed off" on the disease. Soon, people thought "they are bad" about *anyone* who got the virus.

Finally, people just naturally *want* to believe there must be something "bad" about people who get AIDS; thinking so helps them feel they are not likely to get the disease themselves. Treating people with AIDS like "outsiders" calms some people's anxieties, by helping them feel more like "insiders," people who are "good" and therefore must be "safe" from the ailment they fear so much.

Living with AIDS means living with fears about one's health, with the concerns and reactions—good or bad—of one's family and friends, with possible hostility from strangers, and with the constant stress of being ill or trying to maintain one's health. It means working hard to keep on feeling like a good person when others may assume you are a bad person. In David's case it means facing an uncertain future for himself while continuing to work for the healthy future of other young adults. For Luis it means trying to help people exchange unrealistic fears for realistic thoughts and actions—about AIDS and people who have the virus.

As David mentioned, to try to make his own future more secure, he takes a lot of medicines. Some are intended to prevent AIDS-related infections; others are to treat infections he already has. Some—vitamins, minerals, and food supplements—improve his nutrition, providing him enough energy to fight off ailments as well as to work and enjoy life. Some slow the growth of the virus itself, although there is as yet no drug that can stop it or get rid of it.

The medical treatment of AIDS and AIDS-related illnesses can be complex; at present, it is also frustrating. No cure for AIDS has been found, and there is no vaccine to protect people against it.

But the medical fight against AIDS is progressing: as doctors and scientists hunt for ways to battle the disease, they have learned more about viruses and the ways they attack the body, about the immune system, and about new medicines than anyone would have dreamed of ten years ago. And they have found new ways to fight illnesses that afflict people with the virus, so longer lives are possible in many cases.

In chapter five, we will examine some of the main weapons in this ongoing battle for life—the medical war against AIDS—and talk further with the young adults whose bodies have become a battleground.

FIVE

FIGHTING AGAINST AIDS

"I hate my AZT," says Jim S. of the drug he takes every four hours to slow the growth of the AIDS virus in his body. "First of all, it makes me feel sick to my stomach. Often it gives me a headache. It's a constant drag having to remember when to take it, and how many I've already taken. And then because it's every four hours, I have to carry it with me everywhere. I feel like it's always on me, not just with me but *on* me."

It's not just the physical effects of the medicine he dislikes. "They're so expensive, I have to be very careful not to lose them. On top of that, I'm self-conscious about taking them. I feel that if anyone sees me take these, they'll know I have AIDS. Of course I know nobody is really watching me, or would know what I am taking, but I feel as if they might be."

One of Jim's friends, himself diagnosed with the virus and taking AZT, came to Jim's hospital room to show him the capsules soon after Jim learned he would have to begin taking the drug. "It helped me when he did that," Jim says. "To show it to me, so it seemed real and yet not so terrible." He shrugs. "I've only been taking it for a couple of months. People who have been on it longer say you get used to it. I hope they're right."

David Kamens, who takes eighty pills a day and has been on anti-AIDS drugs for several years, thinks Jim will get used to taking a lot of medicine. "Taking pills, it becomes part of your life," he says. "You know you have to take them, so you take them."

Both young men realize that compared with people who got AIDS in the early part of the epidemic, they are relatively fortunate. Of the more than 170,000 who have contracted the virus in the United States since 1981, more than 110,000 have died—most not from the virus itself but of infections and cancers their bodies couldn't fight off.

Christina Lewis, whom we'll meet more fully in Chapter 6, says the medical routine she must follow to stay healthy is difficult. "It's very stressful, almost like a full-time job. I'm taking a medicine called Bactrim to prevent pneumonia, and acyclovir for another infection I had. I have to get vitamin shots; they help my energy level, and they also seem to improve some troubles I've been having with my memory. I visit the doctor regularly, and I have blood tests done. When you have this virus, there's just so much work involved in taking care of yourself."

The virus that causes AIDS is still incurable. Once a person has it, there is no way—no drug, no surgery, no treatment—to get rid of it. Only one drug, zidovudine (called AZT for short) has been approved by the United States Food and Drug Administration as safe and effective for slowing the growth of the virus that causes AIDS. It was first developed as an anti-cancer drug in the 1960s by the chemist Jerome Horwitz of the Michigan Cancer Foundation. AZT turned out not to work against cancer. But in 1987, Dr. Margaret Fischl of the University of Miami School of Medicine began trying the drug on people whose immune systems had already been damaged by the virus. By July 1989 it was obvious that AZT was helping patients who had early symptoms of AIDS. In fact, AZT worked so well that Fischl stopped the test (which involved giving some patients a dummy pill, rather than the real thing) so all in the test group could enjoy the benefits of receiving AZT. The drug was not a "magic bullet" against AIDS, but it was a lot better than nothing.

Another study, by Paul Volberding of San Francisco General Hospital, had even more far-reaching results. By 1989 it showed that the drug could not only help people with AIDS symptoms; it could also keep infected people who did not yet have any symptoms from becoming ill. It is not yet known how long AZT can postpone symptoms in people with the virus, but Secretary of Health and Human Services Louis Sullivan said the drug represented a "milestone in the battle to change AIDS from a fatal disease to a treatable one."

AZT works by keeping the virus from multiplying inside a cell. It can do so because AZT contains a compound much like one the virus uses when it is taking over a cell's reproductive processes. But the AZT compound is not *exactly* like the one the virus needs, so when the virus tries to use it the reproduction of the virus is stopped.

Unfortunately, that's not all AZT does in the human body: it also kills bone-marrow cells, which are the body's supplier of red blood cells. So it can cause severe, even fatal anemia. It is toxic to the liver, the organ that filters a variety of harmful substances from the blood; liver damage can also be fatal. It causes a number of milder, but still very disagreeable side effects: nausea, vomiting, and headaches, among others.

Approximately 50 percent of people with severe symptoms of AIDS must stop taking AZT because of the drug's side effects. Worst of all, even in people who don't experience side effects, AZT eventually stops working against the virus, as over a time that can be as short as six months the virus develops *resistance* (it becomes able to "work around" the reproductive roadblock set up by the drug and can multiply inside the cells again). Because AZT is so toxic and does not work forever, new drugs continue to be sought and tested.

A drug called dideoxyinosine (ddI for short), also developed by chemist Jerome Horwitz but possibly less toxic than AZT, blocks the reproduction of the virus much as AZT does. It does not attack the bone marrow and so does not cause anemia. But it has toxic effects on the pancreas, and inflammation of this organ can be fatal. And it can cause painful damage to nerves. Still, people with advanced AIDS—and even some in the early stages of the ailment—feel that ddI may offer them hope.

"I hope to begin taking ddI instead of AZT," says Jim. He doesn't want to wait until AZT damages his liver or blood supply. He knows that although ddI is not yet approved by the Food and Drug Administration for use against AIDS, it is being tested on people right now by a few physicians who have government approval to do so. Jim hopes to get into one of the test groups.

A substance called alpha interferon is showing promise in some people with the AIDS virus. Interferons are substances the body makes to help fight infections; to fight the virus causing a cold, for instance, interferon spurs destruction of infected cells and causes uninfected ones to make antiviral proteins. "If I were infected," says Dr. Mathilde Krim, a prominent AIDS expert, "I'd treat myself with AZT and alpha interferon." But interferon has its own serious side effects, including anemia, fever, chills, loss of appetite, and potentially fatal heart or breathing abnormalities.

"The government has to speed up the approval for new drugs," says David Kamens, "especially the ones that have already been tested in other countries." He's referring to the lengthy tests the Food and Drug Administration requires before allowing a new drug to be prescribed by American physicians. While people with AIDS are waiting for the FDA to finish testing new anti-AIDS drugs, many of those people are dying. They say they would be willing to take the risks some new drugs pose if they could only be allowed to try them.

Some drugs fight the infections and cancers people with AIDS get, rather than fighting the AIDS virus itself. The virus can damage body organs on its own, but much of the sickness and death it causes are from "opportunistic" ills. (An opportunistic infection is one that can attack the body only when its defenses are lowered for some other reason, such as AIDS.)

They include thrush, which David Kamens now has, and shingles, which caused Ryan White a great deal of pain. They also include pneumocystis pneumonia, the infection that put Jim in the hospital. Even today, with better treatment available, the problems these infections pose have not been entirely solved: 10 to 20 percent of people with pneumocystis pneumonia still die of the disease, for instance. In those who do survive, the infection often comes back. This is because drugs cannot kill every one of the infecting organisms, and in people with AIDS the immune system often cannot fight off even the few surviving germs; once the medicine is stopped, the infection can "blossom" again.

Cytomegalovirus, the infection that afflicted David when he first learned he had AIDS, is a common virus that more than half of all healthy adults have had: it spreads in a variety of ways and causes symptoms like those of mononucleosis. A person who gets this virus carries it in a "quiet phase" forever: it causes no symptoms, probably because the immune system keeps it at low levels of activity. But in a person with AIDS, the immune system can't control cytomegalovirus. The organism can invade and kill the tissues of the eye, causing blindness in about 7 percent of AIDS patients. Or it can infect the digestive tract, which it does in about 5 percent of AIDS patients, causing pain, bleeding, and even death.

Those are only a few of the serious viral and fungal ills that afflict people whose immune systems are damaged by the AIDS virus. In late stages of AIDS, bacterial infections also begin to overwhelm the person's body as the immune sys-

tem can no longer cope with even these relatively less fero-
cious germs. Meanwhile a variety of cancers rarely seen in
people with healthy immune systems also attack people with
AIDS. Perhaps the best known is Kaposi's sarcoma, a cancer
20,000 times more likely to strike people with AIDS than
people with healthy immune systems.

Attacking the lining of blood-vessel walls, Kaposi's sarcoma starts by causing purple skin blotches. Eventually it can
spread through the body, causing serious illness and finally
death. It is treated with radiation to kill malignant cells near
the surface of the body, or with anti-cancer drugs such as
vinblastine if the cancer has spread inwardly. Such treatments usually only slow the spread of the sarcoma, however,
and the drug treatment can have serious side effects, sometimes making the patient less able to fight off other infections. Finding an effective cure for the cancer requires
finding its cause, which is still not known.

Meanwhile the young adults interviewed for this book
keep taking a wide range of expensive, unpleasant treatments that don't always work very well and that often have
side effects ranging from merely disagreeable to the truly
life-threatening. Jim, having survived his first bout with
pneumocystis pneumonia, is still trying to get over the large,
painful cold sore on his lip; he also has an infected ulcer on
one of his tonsils. Dawn says she gets very sick about once a
year; last year she had pneumonia. David gets sick with one
thing after another and must also combat drug side effects so
serious that he's had to be hospitalized for them more than
once. Christina continues her very rigorous medical routine.
And a number of other young adults who wanted to be inter-

viewed for this book were not able to do so: before we could schedule a time to get together they became ill and were simply too sick to talk.

To some, fighting against AIDS means giving money for more education and research; to others it means speaking or writing on the disease, to help people understand it and avoid getting it. For doctors, fighting AIDS means trying to help those who have it, and to scientists the battle means searching for causes and cures as well as for an effective vaccine against the virus that causes AIDS. For those who are not infected, fighting AIDS also means avoiding risky behaviors so as to avoid getting the virus: never sharing hypodermic needles, and never having unsafe sex.

But for the people who have AIDS, fighting it means fighting for life every day: against the virus itself, against infections and cancers, against the side effects of the very medicines they need to take. It means fighting the worry that next time they get sick, the medicine might not work. It means knowing that many others have died of the disease they battle, not ignoring that fact, yet finding the strength to keep up their hopes. In the next chapter we'll hear what they say about how others can avoid what's happened to them.

SIX

AN OUNCE OF PREVENTION

"**D**eciding not to use condoms when I had sex was a stupid decision," says nineteen-year-old Krista Blake, who became infected with the virus that causes AIDS via unsafe sex at age sixteen. "And that stupid decision is what's probably going to kill me."

Krista, an honest, realistic person who minces no words when she talks about AIDS, got the virus from a boy her own age in her own small town in Ohio. Still living with her parents, putting off her planned marriage because of uncertainty about her health and about how she will pay for her medical care, Krista has had serious side effects from the medicines she must take.

"Once I was hospitalized because I had so few red blood cells, my body couldn't function. Another time I had to be quarantined [to stay home and avoid being around other people] to avoid catching infections, when my immune system was really low."

The drugs she needs are not only toxic to her body, but unpleasant: "Breathing pentamadine mist to prevent pneumonia is like breathing diesel fumes," Krista says, and drinking ddI, an experimental anti-viral drug, is like drinking "half a cup of water with fifty cups of sugar in it. It's disgusting-tasting and I take it twice a day. I try to wash it down really fast with something else."

Meanwhile, she knows she could become ill at any time and that her life is likely to be shortened by the virus. She also knows there is no cure and no vaccine against it.

"That's the simple reality," she says. "You might just as well face it." Krista spends much of her time speaking to other teens about her experience, and about the only real weapon there is againt AIDS: not getting it in the first place.

"If I had known when I was sixteen what I know now," she says, "I'd have done everything in my power to avoid getting the virus even if it meant never having sex in my whole life. I mean that. Whatever it took, I'd have done. And I'd definitely have insisted on using a condom when I had sex, no matter who it was with, no matter what they said, every time. Every single time."

Krista's experience shows that having sex without using a condom, even with a classmate or good friend, is risky. She had asked her boyfriend flat out if he had the virus, because she knew he was a hemophiliac and he might have contracted it from the blood products he took to treat that ailment.

"But he lied to me," she says. "He knew he had the virus when we had sex, but he told me he didn't have it. I don't know why he did that; I don't know if he was denying the fact that he had it to himself, or what. I don't justify what he did, and I don't condemn it. It's not for me to judge him. But that is what happened. And if I had insisted on a condom, it wouldn't have happened."

Peter Zamora is another nineteen-year-old who got the virus through unsafe sex when he was sixteen. A year later, Peter got the first hint that he was infected—a hint that terrified him. "I found out after I gave blood in a blood drive at my high school. The Red Cross sent me a letter. They didn't mention AIDS, just said that one of the tests they did on my blood came back positive. But because I had had unsafe sex, AIDS was the first thing I thought of. For six months I was so afraid that I didn't tell anyone; I just threw away the letter and tried to put it out of my mind. I didn't even want to think about having sex either. I was afraid I had it, and afraid I'd give it to someone else."

Then something happened that changed Peter's attitude: he fell in love. "I met one special person who I wanted to have a relationship with, so we both went to get tested so we'd know we were safe having sex with each other. I was still putting the Red Cross letter out of my mind. But in my heart I knew mine was going to be positive, so when the doctor told me I did have the virus I just said 'okay,' and left, like I was feeling all right about it."

Then, Peter says, "I just walked out on the sidewalk, alone. But when I got in the car I started crying. What would my family say? What was going to happen to me? Was I going to die? Was I going to get sick and have a lot of pain? What would happen to my new relationship? Would I lose the person I loved? I was completely overwhelmed with feelings: fear, sadness, anger, uncertainty, so many things. I cried so hard all the way home, I don't even know how I got there."

Two years later, Peter has had only one AIDS-related health problem: a very painful case of shingles. This was treated with medication and now he has recovered from it. He has told his family and friends, and all of them stuck by him, even though it was hard for them at first.

"My older sister was a little afraid for her kids," Peter says, "and asked me if there were any precautions she needed to take so they wouldn't get the virus from me. But after I explained that you can't get it by being around a person, hugging them, and so on, she felt better. She understood that."

Peter's father is among his strongest supporters, although it was hard for them both at first. The family immigrated to the United States from Cuba eleven years ago, and in their culture talking about sex or about AIDS and other sexually transmitted diseases is not considered proper. Peter's father was also very worried about his son.

"When I first talked to him about it, I behaved stronger than I felt," Peter says. "I didn't want to show him how I was really feeling." Today, however, Peter's father is proud of the way his son is handling the situation, of Peter's openness and his work to educate others.

Peter knows he may not always feel as well as he does now, but he takes one day at a time: he exercises, eats healthful foods, tries to stay in good shape and enjoy his life. He is an excellent dancer and has won trophies for ballroom dancing, especially salsa. He spends a lot of time volunteering at a Miami AIDS support center called Body Positive, which offers a range of activities for people who have the virus that causes AIDS or who are affected by it. "It's a great place: we have a gym, a dance floor, aerobics classes, meditation, a theater group, a living room with a TV for people to just relax. I love it."

He also talks to a lot of young adults, trying to prevent them from contracting the virus themselves. "There's a myth in the schools that *everyone* is having sex," he says, "especially among the boys. But that's not true. So I tell people, if you are not having sex because you're not ready, or you're waiting for one special person, or because it's against your religion, or you don't want to disappoint your parents— whatever the reason you're not having sex, that's okay. It's perfectly fine not to be having sex at all."

He goes on: "But if you're having sex now or think you might, then make your decision responsibly. You don't want to go through what I've gone through, believe me. Same with illegal drugs. I certainly don't recommend people use them. Myself, I avoid all drugs. I don't want to take even medically prescribed drugs unless they are really necessary for my health. I take vitamins and that's it. But to people who are using IV drugs now or who think they might, I say this: there are ways to use drugs so that at least you won't get AIDS. It's your life, you know? And just because you're using drugs doesn't mean you don't have the right to avoid getting AIDS. You have the right to protect yourself, and the way to do that is to find out *how* to protect yourself, and do it."

Christina Lewis, another young adult working to educate people about AIDS, was nineteen when she learned she had been infected with the virus two years earlier. She believes she got the virus from a boy whom she dated only once, didn't know well, and never saw again. But on that date, he forced her to have sex with him.

"It was date rape," she says, "but you know, if he hadn't raped me, I might have gone out with him again and I might have had sex with him at some time. So the rape was kind of beside the point as far as the disease goes, because I could have gotten the virus without being raped."

Christina feels that way because she was not in the habit of practicing safer sex. So even if she had willingly had sex with the boy she would not have insisted he use a condom. "At the time I just didn't think AIDS could be a problem for me; neither did my friends. I thought I was being responsible by being on the birth control pill to avoid pregnancy, so I wasn't insisting on condoms when I had sex. I wasn't aware of the danger the virus posed to me personally. It was something that happened to other people, but not to people like me. Only later I found out that it could happen to me—and that it had."

Today, Christina says, she too spends most of her time speaking to other teens about what's happened to her, in hopes of keeping it from happening to someone else. She also arranges for other teens with the virus to speak about their experiences.

"All I can say is, don't flush the future years of your life down the toilet," Christina states. "It's so easy to keep them but you can't get them back once they're gone. I thought I had time, years and years of time, and now it turns out that maybe I don't. And I'm finding more and more teens who have the virus, too, and it's scary. I don't want this to happen to my friends. I don't want this to happen to my generation. I don't want it to happen to anyone. But it *can* happen—to us, to you and me."

One after another, in fact, all the young adults interviewed for this book said the very same things about the way they became infected, whether it was through unsafe sex or sharing needles: I didn't realize the danger. I didn't think my partner would lie to me. I thought it only happened in cities, or to older people, or to drug addicts. I didn't know it could happen to teenagers. The person I had sex with looked so healthy, or I'd known him or her all my life. The person I shared a needle with swore he had never done it before, and I hadn't either, so I thought we were safe. I just didn't think it could happen to me, they all say.

"But if you think it can't happen to *you*," Krista Blake adds, "all you have to do is take a look at me. I was in the National Honor Society, editor of the school newspaper, a basic girl next door living in a small town in the middle of nowhere. And I wasn't doing anything different from what lots of people do."

Krista pauses. "Look," she says, "I knew lots of people who were also having unsafe sex. I worried about getting pregnant, and in that department, I squeaked by: I never got pregnant. But in the most important squeak of my life I didn't squeak by. I relied on luck, and my luck ran out. And if it can happen to me, you'd better believe it can happen to anybody."

How can a person protect herself or himself from becoming infected with the virus that causes AIDS? By *completely* avoiding the two main ways of contracting the virus: unsafe sex, and blood-to-blood contacts such as needle sharing. Avoiding these risky behaviors keeps a person from coming in contact with AIDS.

The only way to be *absolutely* sure of not contracting the virus through sexual contact is to avoid certain kinds of sexual activity altogether. The kinds of sexual activity that can pass the virus from one person to another are:

• Sexual intercourse, in which the male's penis enters the female's vagina, especially if he ejaculates ("comes") inside her body.

• Any sex acts, either between two males or between a male and female, in which one person's penis enters the other person's rectum.

• Sex acts in which one person's mouth comes in contact with the other person's penis, rectum, or vagina.

• Deep kissing ("French kissing") *may* be able to spread the virus if one of the people has cuts, sores, or other breaks in the skin inside the mouth.

In short, it doesn't matter who the people are or what their gender is: what matters is the kind of sexual activity they are having. Having the kinds of sex that can spread the virus but taking steps to protect oneself from contracting AIDS via sexual contact is called practicing "safer sex." It is not called "safe sex" because the virus-preventing methods are not foolproof. That is why avoiding the activities is the only *sure* prevention.

The methods of practicing "safer sex" to lower (but not to eliminate) the risk of getting AIDS are these:

Any time a male's penis enters the body of anyone else, whether the other person is male or female, the male must wear a latex condom, preferably one containing the substance *nonoxynol-9*. A condom is a thin sheath that covers the entire length of the penis; the substance nonoxynol-9 is a chemical that kills sperm, the cells that combine with an egg to produce an embryo.

A condom protects a person in two ways: first, by keeping the skin of the penis from coming in contact with any tiny sores or breaks in the other person's skin, it protects the person who is wearing it from contracting AIDS.

Second, when the person wearing the condom ejaculates ("comes"), the condom keeps the semen from contacting the other person's skin. This protects the other person from any virus that might be in the semen. A condom also protects the other person from virus that might be in tiny scratches or sores on the penis. So using a condom every time a male's penis enters another person's body—whether it enters that person's mouth, vagina, or rectum—protects both people from contracting the virus. Not using a condom—even just one time—exposes both partners to potential infection.

Some facts about condoms: Latex condoms protect against the virus better than those made of other materials. Condoms that contain nonoxynol-9 protect against accidental pregnancy better than ones that don't contain this substance. To be effective, a condom should be new, because old ones can become brittle or broken. Condoms are not reusable; use a new condom every time. No one needs a prescription to buy condoms. You can simply walk into a drugstore, convenience store, or anywhere else they are sold and buy them. To be effective, condoms must be worn correctly. Read the instructions in the package and follow them exactly. After use, the condom should be removed and disposed of properly. If you are going to have sex again right away, use a new condom; don't just leave the first one on.

Although condoms are significantly effective in blocking the virus, they can leak, break, slide off, or be defective. But for young men *and* young women who are sexually active or who think they might be going to have sex with someone soon, condoms are *much* better than nothing.

For a sexually active person, carrying a supply of condoms is a mark of maturity and responsibility. And using them—every single time—is an act of love, both for oneself and for one's partner. After all, why would you want to make love with someone who didn't care about your life, health, and future? And conversely, if you don't care about the other person's life and health, their ability to have a future, why should they want to make love with you?

Sex acts involving contact between one person's mouth and the other person's vagina or rectum can also be made safer. A latex glove, finger cot (a latex sheath), or a latex condom not containing spermicide can be placed over the tongue. Or the woman's genitals can be shielded by a device called a rubber dam; it is a thin sheet of latex that blocks the virus, which might otherwise spread from vaginal fluids into small cuts in the skin of a person's mouth or tongue, or from breaks in the skin of the tongue, lips, or the mouth to the fragile tissues of the vagina.

There are, in addition, a whole range of sexual activities that really are "safe sex," not "safer sex," because they do not spread the virus: they include kissing, hugging, petting, massage, masturbation (unless there are sores, cuts, or broken skin on the hands, or on the genitals), and any other contact that involves only the *outside* of the body. So it is possible to have a sexual relationship without doing any of the activities that can pose a risk of AIDS to either partner, and this is the "absolutely safe" way to have a sexual relationship.

Besides sexual contact, the other main way a person can become infected with the virus that causes AIDS is by blood-to-blood contact: for instance, via needle-sharing. One main reason that people share hypodermic needles is to inject illegal drugs such as heroin, amphetamines, or cocaine. Sharing works, cookers, or cotton can spread the virus, too. If you possibly can, stop using injected drugs. If you try to stop and can't, help is available. Hotlines you can call for help are listed in the back of this book. And, most important, never share hypodermic needles with anyone for any reason.

Besides the drugs we commonly think of as "illegal," there is another illicit drug young adults may share needles in order to use: steroids. These are drugs that cause a person to gain weight and size; athletes sometimes inject them in hopes of improving their performance in sports. Bodybuilders may use them to gain muscle mass. A number of professional athletes have been disqualified from competition in recent years as a result of their use of these dangerous, illegal substances.

Steroids can pose many dangers to a person. They can cause liver damage, damage to the reproductive system, and harm to a person's mind. They have even been linked with some suicides because of their effects on the emotions and on thinking and reasoning. But sharing needles to inject them poses yet another, grimmer danger: the chance of getting AIDS from the shared needle.

It is ironic that in their quest for stronger bodies, some young adults may be losing their futures entirely. If a person is using steroids—or injecting any other drugs—for any reason other than because a doctor has prescribed them, he or she should stop. Failing that, he or she should never share the needle used to inject drugs. Counselors who try to help drug addicts, and who know that many addicts will share needles despite warnings about AIDS, teach them to clean their needles and other drug equipment with bleach and water. But the best thing to do is not to inject any illegal drugs at all.

Any needle, not just a drug needle, can transmit the virus that causes AIDS if someone who is infected uses it and then shares it with another person. A needle used to pierce ears, for instance, can transmit the virus unless it is boiled, cleaned with bleach, or otherwise sterilized. Needles used for acupuncture (a method of pain relief that involves inserting needles into special areas of the skin) can transmit the virus unless properly cleaned between patients. Tattoo needles can spread the virus; unless they are sterilized between customers they can be very dangerous. The reason is that some drug addicts get tattoos to cover their "tracks," the marks left by the injections of illegal drugs. And because many addicts are infected with the AIDS virus, needles used on them may carry it to others unless the needles are fully sterilized.

To avoid the risk of AIDS, ear-piercing should be done only by a doctor, nurse, or other health-care professional who uses a new needle for each patient. Acupuncture should be done only by licensed health-care professionals whose premises and equipment are clean. Tattoos should be done only by persons licensed to do so, whose shops are inspected and certified by the local health department or other health regulating authority.

To sum up, AIDS is not curable. In June 1991, Dr. Robert R. Redfield of the Walter Reed Army Institute of Research in Rockville, Maryland, announced that he and his team had developed a new vaccine. It seemed to help some people who were already infected to fight off the virus. But the vaccine, made by a company called MicroGeneSys, had not yet shown long lasting benefits. It was expected that at least several years of work might still be needed to see if the new vaccine could really help people with AIDS.

So prevention is your best bet. Practicing safer sex and avoiding other blood-to-blood contacts are the ways to reduce your risk of acquiring the virus that causes AIDS. Of course, it's easy to talk about the ways of protecting oneself from the virus, but sometimes it's hard to do them. A boy might refuse to wear a condom. A girl or boy might be too embarrassed to suggest it. A young adult who wants to keep his or her friends might agree to share a hypodermic needle for fear of being called "chicken," or left out of the group. There are all kinds of pressures that can tempt any person to skip the safety measures "just this once."

But, says David Kamens, "You have the absolute right to make choices that you can live with. You are a valuable person, someone who really matters in this world, and you have the right to take care of yourself. So you don't have to ask anyone else's permission to make the healthy decisions that will protect your own life. You are important and you *have* the right. Life is a beautiful thing, you know? A very beautiful, precious thing. I've learned that now. I just hope other teens won't have to learn it the way I learned it."

Luis Q. sums it up even more succinctly. When asked to comment on the possible embarrassment a teenager might face when buying a condom for the first time, refusing to give in to peer-pressure to use drugs or have sex, or insisting that a condom be used when someone does have sex, his answer was short and to the point. Said Luis, "I'd rather be embarrassed than dead."

SEVEN

MY
FUTURE
WITH
AIDS

"**M**y fiancé was the first person I told after I learned I had the virus," says nineteen-year-old Krista. "And it wasn't hard to be honest with him about it. The hard part was telling him that I was going to die. I mean, sure, everybody dies sometime. But I'm not going to live as long as most people do. A lot of people see my ability to say that I'm going to die as giving up. But it's not giving up, it's just facing reality."

For Krista and other young adults infected with the virus

that causes AIDS, "facing reality" means facing some unpleasant possibilities. Statistics on what can happen to people who
have the virus or will get it are for the most part extremely
grim: The CDC estimates that by 1993, 390,000 to 480,000
Americans will be ill and 285,000 to 340,000 will have died
of the disease. In March 1991, the CDC estimated that about
1 million people in the United States had already been infected with the virus; of these it was estimated that perhaps
130,000 are between the ages of thirteen and twenty-one. A
study by the National College Health Association estimates
that among college students alone, 35,000 people may be infected.

Just how bad an AIDS epidemic can be is shown by the
situation in some parts of Africa, where health care and AIDS
education are scarce. In Abidjan, the capital of the Ivory
Coast, for example, AIDS is the leading cause of death among
men and the second leading cause of death among women.
Dr. James Chin of the World Health Organization estimates
that by the year 2000, 40 million people worldwide will
carry the virus, 10 million will be ill, and 10 million children
will be orphaned as a result of the disease.

Of people in the United States aged thirteen to nineteen
already diagnosed with the disease, approximately 40 percent are thought to have acquired the virus via unsafe sex.
About 12 percent may have become infected through IV
drug use. About 7 percent could have become infected
through blood transfusions that carried the virus, and 30
percent through blood products used to treat hemophilia.
About 4 percent of young infected people used IV drugs *and*
had unsafe sex; it's not known by which route those people
became infected. And in a very few cases the way a young

person became infected is not known: some people refuse to talk about it, a few don't tell the truth about the risky behaviors they may have engaged in, some simply have no apparent risk factors, and some become too ill to talk to doctors before the way they acquired the virus can be learned.

Because AIDS has been under study for only a little more than ten years, scientists do not know if everyone who has the virus will develop symptoms of the disease. But so far about three in ten people who have the virus have become ill within five years of infection; five of ten have become ill within seven years. Scientists believe that everyone infected will eventually become ill; only time will tell if this is true.

The amount of time it takes an infected person to develop serious symptoms of AIDS varies widely; some people—especially small children and infants—can die within a few months, while others, most of them adults, take years to develop symptoms. A few infected adults have lived for as long as ten years without becoming ill at all, but "long-time survivors" are exceptional.

It is not yet known what pattern the infection will take in teenagers—whether infected teens will get sick quickly, like children, or more slowly, like adults. To get this information medical studies will have to be done. But once a person of any age begins getting the serious AIDS-related ailments, his or her likely life span shortens dramatically. Adults who survive an attack of the AIDS-related pneumonia *Pneumocystis carinii,* for instance, may live an average of only three more years, even when given the best medical treatment now available; again, it is not yet known what the life spans of teens and younger adults who get such illnesses may turn out to be.

How do young adults face the possibility of serious illness or early death? How do they confront what the future may hold for them? The psychiatrist Elizabeth Kübler-Ross originated the idea, now widely accepted, that almost all people with a potentially fatal illness go through a series of steps in handling the reality of their condition.

The first step is often *denial:* simply not being able to believe that it is true. Peter Zamora was seventeen when he learned he had the virus that causes AIDS. But he denied his condition for six months, throwing away the letter that told him about it, refusing to think about it. Others tell themselves the test results are wrong, the blood samples got mixed up—anything other than that they have the virus. Once they do believe it, most people are frightened.

"At first," says Christina, "I was just so scared I couldn't think. I thought, 'Oh, my God, I'm gonna die.' But then I went out and learned all I could about this disease." For Christina, as for most of the young adults interviewed for this book, finding out as much as possible about the virus and their condition gave them a sense of control. Knowledge did not erase their fears, but it did make them seem more manageable. In Christina's case, knowing more meant finding out her situation was indeed very serious, but perhaps not as totally bleak as she had feared in the beginning.

"I learned I had the virus from a letter," she says. "I had donated blood, and then gone to France on a month's vacation. So when the Red Cross had tested my blood and it came back positive, they couldn't reach me by telephone, which is I assume why they sent me a letter about it. When I got home from vacation and picked up my mail, there it was. I opened it in the car, and all I saw was the word AIDS. And I just freaked out."

When she reached her apartment, her roommate was home. "Thank God he was there," she says. "I just threw the letter at him, and said 'Read this!' I was crying, and my roommate was French so he didn't understand what the letter said. I said 'It means I have AIDS!' But once he did understand, he just sat me down and said, 'Okay, now, we need to see what we should do.' I don't know what I would have done without him being there, I was just so freaked out."

Not all Christina's friends reacted quite as calmly as her roommate did, partly because some received information about AIDS that was not accurate. For example: "That night, right after I got the letter, I had friends coming over, and I told them I'd just learned I had the virus. And this one friend and I had shared an Epilady—one of those gadgets that plucks the hair out of your legs? Well, she was concerned about that, so she asked my doctor if she could get AIDS from sharing the Epilady. And he told her she should get tested. Which was totally wrong, you can't get the virus that way. There's no blood contact there. But she was worried for a while, because of the wrong information he told her."

Christina herself also got some inaccurate information from this doctor, who did not understand AIDS. "He basically told me that I had only about a year and a half to live. That was not only wrong, it was also damaging. Because if you believe it, that's how long you'll live. Then you'll give up and die. This doctor has since been fired by the health department. But after I got more and better information and thought about what I had learned, I realized what he told me couldn't be right. Also, I found out there were things I could do, I wasn't going to die *tomorrow*. People like me who have the virus but no symptoms have a longer life span than I thought. I began to realize I didn't have to give up right off the bat. And I haven't.''

Still, she does not ignore the fact that the virus often causes fatal illness—that it may shorten her own life just as it has shortened others' lives. "I wish," she says, "that I'd gotten it when I was thirty, not when I was a teenager. Then I'd have had so much more time—to finish my education, to get more skills, everything I want to do. I mean, people who don't have the virus have all kinds of things they're planning to do, hopes for their future, things they want to get out of life and things they want to contribute. I have all those things, too. The only difference is, I may not get the time to do them."

Telling her family she was infected was so difficult for Christina that she ended up not being able to do it herself. "I kept trying, but every time I was about to tell them, my heart started pounding and my palms started sweating. I finally asked my brother to tell them, and he did. At first, of course, they were completely distraught. Fortunately, by that time I had gained the information I needed and had gotten over my own first shock and fright. Otherwise we'd have all been terribly upset at the same time. They've been wonderfully supportive to me, but some people haven't been helpful to them, unfortunately, especially some people where my father was working."

The problem at her father's job had to do with Christina's health insurance, which was provided through her father's policy. Because AIDS-related illnesses are so expensive to treat, it would have cost the company a lot to continue providing health insurance for Christina. She and her family believe this is why her father, who had previously been promoted regularly, suddenly began getting demoted to lower and lower positions. "At the end," Christina says, "he was just sitting there with a desk, a phone, and nothing to do. Finally they fired him."

Christina's dad doesn't know if he'll be able to get another job, and in a few more months the whole family will be without health insurance. They are pursuing legal remedies to this situation, because it is illegal to fire someone just to get the person or one of his or her family members off a health insurance policy. But so far no solution has been found.

Christina herself was dismissed from the job she held when she first learned she had the virus. "I told them because there was going to be a magazine article about me, so I thought they'd better hear it from me before they read it, or the customers read it. And my manager and everyone I worked with was perfectly fine about it," she says, "but I guess the higher-ups in the company didn't want to deal with me having the virus. I was a hostess in a restaurant; I suppose they thought it would be bad publicity." In that case, however, Christina threatened to sue and was given her job back at once.

Even after the intense early fears have eased somewhat, and as many practical problems—such as jobs and insurance—as possible have been solved, it is not easy to live with the reality of having the virus. Many young adults who cope with their situation by trying to educate others about AIDS say that work helps them—but they still worry about friends and families, especially about their feelings.

"I have spent a lot of time thinking about things that

could happen to me from this virus," says Christina, who was seventeen when she became infected. "But I'm not going to worry about it every day. That is a waste of time, and it's not good for me, either. In a way it's harder for my friends and family: my parents, my brothers, everyone. Because if I go, I'm gone. But they will still have to be here, living with it."

Krista agrees. "I decided very early on that I could either let it get the best of me, or I could get the best of it for as long as I can until I have no control left at all. And I decided I would get the best of it, by going out and educating as many other people as I could, so they wouldn't become infected. For the people close to me, though, when I die, it will be very hard. Because they will have to watch me die. I have a best friend, for instance, and I asked her to be the one who would decide to turn off my life-support systems if that were necessary. But she couldn't answer me. All she could do was cry. Imagine if I were your best friend, how you would feel. Your best friend is dying and all you can do is watch."

Jim S. also thinks about how it would affect those closest to him if he should die, and of how hard it is for them to think that he might. His longtime companion, Art, has told Jim that sometimes when he is by himself he begins to cry. Art worries about what might happen to Jim; he does not want Jim to suffer. But he also worries about what life would be like without Jim, whom he dreads losing. Like anyone else, he hates the thought that the person he loves might die.

"I'm very glad he talks to me about how he feels," says Jim. "And sometimes we talk about the disease on a purely practical level: my medications, or about money, day-to-day things like that. But we also discuss things on a deeper level: what the disease means to our lives together and to the future. And it breaks my heart to hear how sad it makes him sometimes. He doesn't want me to leave him."

Jim worries about his parents, too; he has become closer to them since they learned of his illness, but he feels they do not have anyone to talk to about it. This, he thinks, will make it all the more difficult for them if he should die.

Peter notes that infected people who have no symptoms at all worry about their future, perhaps even as much as people who have already become ill from the virus. "You get a little bump on your skin, or a rash, or a little sore throat, and right away you're thinking 'this might be something, this might be the start of something very bad.' I'm scared of dying, but at this point it's uncertainty, for me, that's so hard to deal with. Will I even reach the age of twenty-one? So I take it a day at a time. If it comes tomorrow, whatever it is, I'll deal with it tomorrow. But it's not here yet." Peter has also found a creative way to use another emotion many young adults with the virus that causes AIDS feel: anger.

Almost everyone who faces having a potentially fatal illness gets angry, as a natural reaction to their situation. They feel hurt and want to hit back at the threat to their lives, and at a world that seems to have wounded them unjustly. They may express their anger toward a doctor, their families and friends, toward a person whom they think may have given them the virus, or toward themselves, by blaming themselves for contracting the virus.

The anger they feel can lead to depression if they turn it inward or don't have anyone with whom they can discuss their feelings. It can make them seem hostile and irritable, causing their loved ones to "back off" from the person—at a time when they want to be close to the person and comfort him or her. But a person feeling such anger needs time and understanding to deal with it. And he or she needs to know that friends and family aren't going to abandon him or her on account of the anger—or on account of the virus.

Eventually the worst of the anger fades in most people. No young adult who was interviewed for this book, for instance, said he or she was still very angry at any specific person, at God, or about their own situation. Most seemed to feel that anger was a waste of time, and they valued their own time too highly to spend much on negative emotions. But Peter has kept some of his anger. He uses it, he says, to keep his energy levels high, so he can keep helping others and educating young adults about AIDS.

"For instance, if I get tired, or I start to wonder why I'm working so hard, why I'm doing this," he says, "I remember how I first felt when I found out I had the virus, or how I feel when a close friend dies of it, or how I feel about the suffering and pain the disease causes. My anger over that, about how senseless it all is, helps me keep going.

"Also," Peter goes on, "I sometimes get angry at society: because there needs to be so much more awareness about AIDS, but there isn't, and also because to a lot of society I have a label: it reads, 'Teenager With AIDS.' I get angry when people don't see beyond the label. Because I am a person, a whole person, and there's much more to me than just 'Teenager With AIDS.' But it is just another thing I have to live with, so when I get angry I use all that anger as fuel to keep me going."

Many people facing a possibly fatal illness enter a stage of bargaining: they may say that if only the virus can be taken away from their bodies, they will "be good," or give up something they enjoy very much, or break all their bad habits, for example.

Dawn Marcal remembers a kind of bargaining she went through, not for her own life, but for her daughter's: "Every night when we were waiting for the test results to come back," she says, "I would go to bed, and I would pray. Please, God, I said, if I do have to have this disease, I can accept that. If I have to die from the disease, I can accept that. But please, God—not my daughter. I love her so much. Please don't let my child have to suffer for my mistakes."

But because the virus that causes AIDS—like other serious illnesses—has nothing to do with whether a person is "good" or "bad," there is no way to bargain away the fact that one has it. And sooner or later, many people facing the possibility of their own deaths leave the bargaining, the anger, and much of their fear behind them. They stop trying to push the disease out of their minds and begin to concentrate on living the lives they do have.

Acceptance of their situation may bring some people with AIDS an unexpected benefit: a new awareness of the value of life and of the really important things in it. No one is ever glad to have the virus that causes AIDS, but almost everyone in this book said they had learned things of great value from what they are going through.

"Before," says Christina, "I didn't really think about how very important my friends and family are to me, and how valuable my time is. I don't waste time anymore. I do the things I want to do in life. And I take care of my relationships: if something does happen to me, I won't feel there's something I haven't done, something I haven't said, with the people who really matter to me. I won't be leaving with that kind of regret."

Agrees Peter, "So many things that used to be important just aren't important to me anymore. A nice car is fine, but it's not really important in my life, for instance. Understanding my own feelings, finding out who I am as a person and what I do want to accomplish, taking care of myself by using energy on things that are worth it, not on trivial things—to me those are the really important things in life now."

Krista's attitude about her town and the people in it is one of the many things that have changed since she learned she had the virus. "I was negative about the town," she says. "I hated it, and I wanted to get away from it so much. But now I wonder, if I'd been anywhere else and this happened to me, would the people have been so supportive, so nonjudgmental? I haven't had any goofy reactions from people here. No hostility, nothing like that. Some people couldn't talk to me at first, but it was only that they felt bad about what had happened to me. They weren't shunning me. They just had to deal with their own sorrow before they could deal directly with me."

"There was a time in my life when I thought everything was so terrible," says Dawn. "And I just couldn't see it getting better. It seemed to me that my life was just so bad, during my teenage years. But now I feel that life is a wonderful thing, and I appreciate living each day." Agrees David, "I can't say life is actually better since I became sick, because of course, it's not. My immune system is pretty much gone, and I get one illness after another. But as far as the way I see life itself, all I can say is, it's like the difference between seeing in black and white, versus seeing life in color. I appreciate all the little things so much more. And I'm really aware that life is very precious."

Christina and Jim had one more comment about living with the virus that causes AIDS: Yes, it's bad. Yes, it can cause very serious illness and death. But don't be so afraid of AIDS that you can't absorb the facts. Don't just "block it out."

"Before I got sick, the very idea of getting AIDS was so terrifying," says Jim, "that I could not even imagine how I would deal with it. And I think a lot of unknown things in life are like that. The imagination of what might happen can be so much worse than the reality of it. I mean, this is not a good thing that's happened. I hope every day that there will be a cure, I'll get the virus out of my body, and be able to go on with my life. But I am dealing with it."

Jim feels that people shouldn't fear the disease so much that they push the thought of it from their minds; doing so would prevent them from acquiring the very information they need to help them avoid contracting the virus themselves. Adds Christina, "It's important to know that it's not the end of the world, even if you find out you have the virus. There are ways to control your life and what happens to your body, at least to a certain extent. You can go and have quite a few good years. I really value the last few years of my life; they've been more incredible than the first ones."

Like Jim, Christina feels that one of the most important things people need to do is stop ignoring AIDS, whether out of fear or for any reason. "We've got to stop thinking this only happens to other people," she says, "because it doesn't. It happens to us."

"I plan on living as long as I can, doing as much as I can

while I'm still alive," says Krista, expressing the determination and spirit all the other interviewed young adults showed in their different ways. "I can't change what is in the past, I can't go back and undo it. But I can refuse to give up until I do run completely out of energy. I can live the best way I can with the amount of life I do have. And that's what I'm going to do."

One after another all the young adults interviewed for this book have had to face a future filled with uncertainty, with the chance of very serious illness or with illnesses already endured, and with the frightening chance that they may not have the long healthy lives uninfected people take for granted.

Dawn has lost her only child, along with her own robust health. Krista has had to postpone her marriage indefinitely. Mike has learned at age fifteen that life may not stretch forever into the future. David has been through numerous painful and dangerous illnesses. Jim has survived one life-threatening bout with pneumonia and seen his life and hopes for future career accomplishments turned upside down. All have had to think about saying good-bye to their loved ones before they thought they would, and about the pain and sorrow they will leave behind if that happens.

So why, in the midst of their own problems, did these young people bother being interviewed for this book? Why did they all spend precious time and energy telling their stories when they could have been doing other things instead? Christina speaks out for the group: "If just one person reads it, and doesn't get AIDS because of it—if just one person's life gets to go on uninterrupted—then it's worth it. Because when you tell people the facts about this virus or what it's like living with it, and about the things that can happen or have happened to you because of it, you always just hope and pray that's what the outcome will be: maybe someone will listen.

"Of course you never know who that someone is, and you never find out, because as a result of their listening to you nothing happens to them. They think about what you have said and avoid risky behaviors. They protect themselves and don't get AIDS, so they never have to go through what you have gone through.

"And that's what I hope," Christina concludes, "that's why I talk about this. By telling about my experience and what has happened to me, maybe I can help save even one person's life, and that one life—just one single life—would make doing it worthwhile to me."

GLOSSARY

AIDS Acquired *I*mmuno-*D*eficiency *S*yndrome, a condition in which the body's immune system has been damaged by a retrovirus, the human immunodeficiency virus, so that it can no longer fight off infections and other illnesses.

ANTIBODIES Particles produced by the immune system to fight off infections.

AZT The brand name for zidovudine, the only U.S.-approved drug that can slow the growth of the virus that causes AIDS in human beings.

CONDOM A thin latex sheath worn on the penis during sexual contact to prevent pregnancy and to lower the risk of getting or spreading the virus that causes AIDS.

DENIAL The condition of refusing to believe that something is true, when in fact it is true.

ELISA Enzyme-Linked Immunosorbent Assay, a test used to determine whether a person's blood contains antibodies against the virus that causes AIDS.

EPIDEMIC A disease that attacks many people over a short period of time.

ESOPHAGUS The tube in the body that carries food from the mouth to the stomach.

FACTOR IV   A medication made from human blood, used to treat hemophilia.

FUNGAL   Caused by an organism that is related to yeasts or molds.

GENERIC   The non-brand name of a drug; common or generally named.

GENDER   The physical maleness or femaleness of an individual.

HEMOPHILIA   An inherited condition in which a person's blood does not clot properly.

HERPES SIMPLEX   The virus that causes "cold sores."

HETEROSEXUAL   A person who is sexually attracted primarily to those of the opposite gender.

HIV   Human immunodeficiency virus, the virus that causes AIDS.

HOMOSEXUAL   A person who is sexually attracted primarily to others of his or her own gender.

HYPODERMIC NEEDLE   The kind of needle that is used to inject drugs.

IMMUNE SYSTEM   The system of the body that fights off illness and infections.

IMMUNODEFICIENCY   A condition in which the immune system has been damaged or destroyed.

IV (INTRAVENOUS) DRUG   A drug that is injected into the bloodstream.

KAPOSI'S SARCOMA A kind of skin cancer that people with AIDS often get.

LATENT PERIOD The time after a person has become infected with the virus that causes AIDS, but before the infection can be detected by blood tests.

NEGATIVE A test result that shows that a person does not have the disease or condition for which he or she is being tested.

OPPORTUNISTIC INFECTION An infection that a person can only get when his or her immune system is not working properly.

PENTAMADINE A medication used to treat or prevent the pneumonia people with AIDS often get.

PNEUMOCYSTIS CARINII The organism that causes the pneumonia people with AIDS often get.

POSITIVE A test result that shows that a person does have the disease or condition for which he or she is being tested.

RESISTANCE The body's ability to fight off disease.

RETROVIRUS A special kind of virus containing the chemical reverse transcriptase, which enables the virus to imitate the cell's instructions for reproducing itself and to become part of the cell. The AIDS virus is a retrovirus.

SAFER SEX Sexual activities that do not involve one person's blood or semen coming into contact with another's uncovered skin.

SEXUALLY TRANSMITTED DISEASE A disease that can be spread by sexual contact.

SIDE EFFECTS   Effects of a medicine other than the effects that are wanted.

STIGMA   An invisible "mark of shame."

STRAINS   Different forms of the same virus.

SYNDROME   A group of symptoms or health problems that go along with an illness.

T-4 CELLS   Cells in the immune system that tell the body to start fighting an illness.

T-8 CELLS   Cells in the immune system that tell the body it can stop fighting an illness.

UNSAFE SEX   Sexual activity in which one person's blood or semen comes into contact with another person's unprotected skin.

VACCINE   A medication generally given to prevent a person from becoming infected with a disease-causing virus, but in the case of AIDS, used experimentally to stimulate the immune system to fight an infection that is already present.

VIRUS   An extremely tiny organism that does nothing but infect cells of other creatures and causes those cells to make more viruses.

WESTERN BLOT   A blood test that can detect antibodies to the virus that causes AIDS; more sensitive than the ELISA test.

ZIDOVUDINE   The generic name for the drug AZT.

FOR MORE INFORMATION AND ASSISTANCE

For information on AIDS testing and counseling, and about AIDS resources in your area:

National AIDS Hotline: 800-342-AIDS
Spanish: 800-344-7432
Deaf Access: 800-243-7889 [TTY]

For additional information on AIDS:

American Red Cross AIDS Education Office
1730 D Street, N.W.
Washington, DC 20006
202-737-8300

Federal Centers for Disease Control
1600 Clinton Road N.E.
Atlanta, GA 30333
404-639-3311

Gay Men's Health Crisis
P.O. Box 274
132 West 24th Street
New York, NY 10011
212-807-6655

National Council of Churches/AIDS Task Force
475 Riverside Drive, Room 572
New York, NY 10115
212-863-2437

National Gay and Lesbian Lifeline
80 Fifth Avenue
New York, NY 10011
212-529-1600

San Francisco AIDS Foundation
25 Van Ness Avenue
San Francisco, CA 94102
415-864-5855

For information on effective use of condoms call the office of Planned Parenthood listed in your local telephone book or:

Planned Parenthood Federation of America, Inc.
810 Seventh Avenue
New York, NY 10019
212-541-7800

For information on hemophilia and AIDS:

Hemophilia Foundation
104 East 40th Street
New York, NY 10016
212-682-5510

For information on sexually transmitted diseases:

National Sexually Transmitted Diseases Hotline
American Social Health Association: 800-227-8922

For information about experimental AIDS treatments:

AIDS Clinical Trials Information Services: 800-874-2572

For help in finding resources and information:

National AIDS Information Clearinghouse
P.O. Box 6003
Rockville, MD 20850
800-458-5231

For information on AIDS throughout the world:

World Health Organization: 202-861-4340

To arrange for a young adult to speak to a school or other group about AIDS, and for information on resources in your area:

National Association of People With AIDS (NAPWA)
1413 K Street, N.W., 10th floor
Washington, DC 20005
202-898-0414

For information on homosexuality or for referral to a local support group:

Parents and Friends of Lesbian and Gay Youth
P.O. Box 27605
Washington, DC 20038
202-638-4200

For information about drug abuse treatment in your area:

Drug Abuse Treatment Information Referral Line:
800-662-HELP

FURTHER READING

Altman, Dennis. *AIDS in the Mind of America.* New York: Doubleday, 1986.

Check, William. *AIDS.* New York: Chelsea House, 1988.

Dwyer, John M. *The Body at War: The Miracle of the Immune System.* New York: New American Library, 1989.

Glaser, Elisabeth, and Laura Palmer. *In the Absence of Angels.* New York: Putnam, 1991.

Hein, Karen, M.D., and Theresa Foy DeGeronimo. *AIDS: Trading Fears for Facts.* Mount Vernon, N.Y.: Consumers Union, 1989.

Kübler-Ross, Elizabeth. *AIDS: The Ultimate Challenge.* New York: Macmillan, 1987.

Landau, Elaine. *We Have AIDS.* New York: Watts, 1990.

LeVert, Suzanne. *AIDS: In Search of a Killer.* New York: Julian Messner, 1987.

Madaras, Lynda. *Lynda Madaras Talks to Teens About AIDS.* New York: Newmarket 1988.

Martelli, Leonard. *When Someone You Know Has AIDS.* New York: Crown, 1987.

Moustafa, Laila, ed. *The AIDS Handbook: A Complete Guide To Education and Awareness.* New York: Designbase Publishing, 1991.

Schilling, Sharon. *My Name is Jonathan and I Have AIDS.* Denver, Colo: Prickly Pair Press, 1989. (Also available in Spanish and Vietnamese)

Shilts, Randy. *And the Band Played On: People, Politics, and AIDS.* New York: St. Martin's, 1987.

United States Public Health Service. *Understanding the Immune System.* Bethesda, Md.: National Institutes of Health, 1988.

White, Ryan, and Ann Marie Cunningham. *Ryan White: My Own Story.* New York: Dial, 1991.

SOURCES

Periodicals

Altman, Lawrence K. "W.H.O. Says 40 Million Will Be Infected With AIDS Virus by 2000." *New York Times,* June 18, 1991.

Aral, Sevgi O., and King K. Holmes. "Sexually Transmitted Diseases in the AIDS Era." *Scientific American,* February 1991, p. 62.

Barnes, Deborah M. "Keeping AIDS Out of the Blood Supply." *Science,* August 1, 1986, p. 514.

Begley, Sharon, Mary Hager, and Larry Wilson. "Desperation Drugs." *Newsweek,* August 7, 1989, p. 48.

Borhek, Mary V. "Helping Gay and Lesbian Adolescents and their Families." *Journal of Adolescent Health Care* 9, No. 2 (1988): 123.

Bower, Bruce. "Teenage Turning Point." *Science News,* March 23, 1991, p. 184.

Brooks-Gunn, J., Cherrie Boyer, and Karen Hein, M.D. "Preventing HIV Infection and AIDS in Children and Adolescents." *American Psychologist,* November 1988, p. 958.

Cowley, Geoffrey, Mary Hager, and Ruth Marshall. "AIDS, The Next Ten Years." *Newsweek,* June 25, 1990, p. 20.

Culliton, Barbara. "Crash Development of AIDS Test Nears Goal." *Science,* September 14, 1984, p. 1128.

De Cock, K. M. et al. "AIDS—The Leading Cause of Death in

the West African City of Abidjan, Ivory Coast." *Science* 249 (17 August 1990): 793.

Dworkin, Peter, and Scott Minerbrook. "The AIDS Threat to Teenagers." *US News & World Report,* October 23, 1989, p. 29.

Ezzell, E. "New Evidence Supports a Cofactor In AIDS." *Science News,* March 2, 1991, p. 133.

Fackelman, K. A. "Early AZT Use Slows Progression to AIDS." *Science News,* August 26, 1989, p. 135.

―――. "Drug Spray Strikes Out In Severe Pneumonia." *Science News,* June 2, 1990, p. 348.

―――. "Data And Dispute Mark AIDS Meeting." *Science News,* June 30, 1990, p. 404.

"Family In AIDS Case Quits Florida Town After House Burns." *New York Times,* August 29, 1987, p. 1.

Flora, June A., and Carl E. Thoresen. "Reducing the Risks of AIDS in Adolescents." *American Psychologist,* November 1988, p. 965.

Freundlich, Naomi, John Carey, and Joan O'C. Hamilton. "AIDS: A Break in the Gloom." *Business Week,* June 25, 1990, p. 22.

Glaser, Elisabeth, and Laura Palmer. "In the Absence of Angels." *People Weekly,* February 4, 1991, p. 85.

Goodman, Elizabeth, M.D., and Alwyn T. Cohall, M.D. "Acquired Immunodeficiency Syndrome and Adolescents." *Pediatrics* 84, No. 1 (July 1989): 36.

Gorman, Christine. "At Last a Sensible AIDS Plan." *Time,* March 7, 1988, p. 58.

Hein, Karen, M.D. "Commentary on Adolescent Acquired Immunodeficiency Syndrome: The Next Wave of the Human Immunodeficiency Epidemic?" *Journal of Pediatrics,* Vol 114 (January 1989): 144.

Hendricks, Melissa. "Two AIDS Drugs May Be Better Than One." *Science News*, September 10, 1988, p. 172.

Herek, Gregory M., and Eric K. Glunt. "An Epidemic of Stigma: Public Reactions to AIDS." *American Psychologist*, November 1988, p. 886.

Hersch, Patricia. "Coming of Age on the City Streets." *Psychology Today*, January 1988, p. 28.

"HIV-Related Beliefs, Knowledge and Behaviors among High School Students." *Clinical Pediatrics* 28 (June 1989): 284.

Horgan, John. "Strength In Numbers: Researchers Begin Combining Compounds to Fight AIDS." *Scientific American*, July 1990, p. 20.

Kiecolt-Glaser, Janice K., and Ronald Glaser. "Psychological Influences on Immunity: Implications for AIDS." *American Psychologist*, November 1988, p. 892.

Koop, C. Everett, M.D. "Surgeon General's Report on Acquired Immune Deficiency Syndrome." U.S. Department of Health and Human Services, 1989.

Krajick, Kevin. "Private Passions, Public Health." *Psychology Today*, May 1988, p. 50.

Manning, D. Thompson, and Paul Bolson. "Teenagers' Beliefs About AIDS Education and Physicians' Perceptions about Them." *Journal of Family Practice* 29, No. 2 (1989): 173.

Mills, John, and Henry Masur. "AIDS-Related Infections." *Scientific American*, August 1990, p. 50.

Monmaney, Terence. "The Return of AZT." *Discover*, January 1990, p. 58.

"Mystery Microbe May Cause AIDS Cancer." *Science News*, March 3, 1990, p. 78.

Palca, John. "Trials and Tribulations of AIDS Testing." *Sci-*

ence, March 23, 1990, p. 1406.

Radetsky, Peter. "Closing In on an AIDS Vaccine." *Discover,* September 1990, p. 70.

Redfield, Robert R., M.D. et al. "A Phase I Evaluation of the Safety and Immunogenicity of Vaccination with Recombinant gp160 in Patients with Early Human Immunodeficiency Virus Infection." *New England Journal of Medicine* 324 (June 13, 1991): 1677.

Remafedi, Gary, M.D. "Preventing the Sexual Transmission of AIDS During Adolescence." *Journal of Adolescent Health Care* 9, No. 2 (1988): 139.

Rivera, Ruben, Jr. *A Basic AIDS/HIV Prevention Education Curriculum.* New Haven: Privately printed, 1988.

Seligman, Jean, and Ruth Marshall. "Checking Up On A Killer." *Newsweek,* June 12, 1989, p. 59.

Silberner, Joanne. "AIDS Blood Test Qualified Success." *Science News,* August 10, 1985, p. 84.

————. "AIDS Blood Screen." *Science News,* July 26, 1986, p. 56.

U.S. Department of Health and Human Services/Centers for Disease Control. *HIV/AIDS Surveillance.* May 1991.

Weiss, Rick. "Improving the AIDS Test." *Science News,* April 2, 1988, p. 218.

————. "AIDS Vaccine: Safe, But Does It Work?" *Science News,* January 19, 1991, p. 38.

BOOKS

Altman, Dennis. *AIDS In the Mind of America.* New York: Doubleday, 1986.

Dalton, Harlon L., Scott Burris, and the Yale AIDS Law Project. *AIDS and the Law: A Guide for the Public.* New Haven: Yale University Press, 1987.

Hein, Karen, M.D., and Theresa Foy DeGeronimo. *AIDS: Trading Fears for Facts.* Mount Vernon, N.Y.: Consumers Union, 1989.

Hippler, Mike. *So Little Time: Essays On Gay Life.* Berkeley, Calif: Celestial Arts Books, 1990.

Kübler-Ross, Elizabeth. *AIDS: The Ultimate Challenge.* New York: Macmillan, 1987.

LeVert, Suzanne. *AIDS: In Search of a Killer.* New York: Julian Messner, 1987.

Shilts, Randy. *And the Band Played On: People, Politics and AIDS.* New York: St. Martin's, 1987.

INDEX

Mary Kittredge is the author of more than a dozen books of non-fiction for young adults, including titles on *Organ Transplants, The Respiratory System, The Senses, First Aid and Emergency Medicine,* and *The Human Body: An Overview.* Her other books include biographies and six mysteries. She was associate editor of the professional journal *Respiratory Care* and for fifteen years was a certified respiratory therapy technician at Yale-New Haven Hospital in New Haven, Connecticut.

Dale C. Garell, M.D. is Executive Associate Dean and Professor of Clinical Family Medicine and Pediatrics at the University of Southern California School of Medicine. From 1978 to 1990 he was medical director of California Children's Services for the County of Los Angeles. He has been a member of the Ad Hoc AIDS Committee of the American Academy of Pediatrics and president of the Society for Adolescent Medicine. In 1989 he served as Co-chair of the Fifth National Pediatric AIDS Conference. Dr. Garell is the general editor of a 79-volume encyclopedia of health for young adults.